NATIONAL ACADEMIES *Sciences Engineering Medicine*

NATIONAL ACADEMIES PRESS
Washington, DC

Methadone Treatment for Opioid Use Disorder

Improving Access Through Regulatory and Legal Change

Lisa Bain, Sheena M. Posey Norris, and Clare Stroud, *Rapporteurs*

Board on Health Sciences Policy

Board on Health Care Services

Health and Medicine Division

Action Collaborative on Countering the U.S. Opioid Epidemic

Proceedings of a Workshop

NATIONAL ACADEMY OF MEDICINE

THE NATIONAL ACADEMIES PRESS 500 Fifth Street, NW Washington, DC 20001

This activity was supported by a contract between the National Academy of Sciences and the Office of National Drug Control Policy, Executive Office of the President (11316021P0001OND). Any opinions, findings, conclusions, or recommendations expressed in this publication do not necessarily reflect the views of any organization or agency that provided support for the project.

International Standard Book Number-13: 978-0-309-69096-6
International Standard Book Number-10: 0-309-69096-X
Digital Object Identifier: https://doi.org/10.17226/26635

This publication is available from the National Academies Press, 500 Fifth Street, NW, Keck 360, Washington, DC 20001; (800) 624-6242 or (202) 334-3313; http://www.nap.edu.

Copyright 2022 by the National Academy of Sciences. National Academies of Sciences, Engineering, and Medicine and National Academies Press and the graphical logos for each are all trademarks of the National Academy of Sciences. All rights reserved.

Printed in the United States of America.

Suggested citation: National Academies of Sciences, Engineering, and Medicine. 2022. *Methadone treatment for opioid use disorder: Improving access through regulatory and legal change: Proceedings of a workshop.* Washington, DC: The National Academies Press. https://doi.org/10.17226/26635.

The **National Academy of Sciences** was established in 1863 by an Act of Congress, signed by President Lincoln, as a private, nongovernmental institution to advise the nation on issues related to science and technology. Members are elected by their peers for outstanding contributions to research. Dr. Marcia McNutt is president.

The **National Academy of Engineering** was established in 1964 under the charter of the National Academy of Sciences to bring the practices of engineering to advising the nation. Members are elected by their peers for extraordinary contributions to engineering. Dr. John L. Anderson is president.

The **National Academy of Medicine** (formerly the Institute of Medicine) was established in 1970 under the charter of the National Academy of Sciences to advise the nation on medical and health issues. Members are elected by their peers for distinguished contributions to medicine and health. Dr. Victor J. Dzau is president.

The three Academies work together as the **National Academies of Sciences, Engineering, and Medicine** to provide independent, objective analysis and advice to the nation and conduct other activities to solve complex problems and inform public policy decisions. The National Academies also encourage education and research, recognize outstanding contributions to knowledge, and increase public understanding in matters of science, engineering, and medicine.

Learn more about the National Academies of Sciences, Engineering, and Medicine at **www.nationalacademies.org**.

Consensus Study Reports published by the National Academies of Sciences, Engineering, and Medicine document the evidence-based consensus on the study's statement of task by an authoring committee of experts. Reports typically include findings, conclusions, and recommendations based on information gathered by the committee and the committee's deliberations. Each report has been subjected to a rigorous and independent peer-review process and it represents the position of the National Academies on the statement of task.

Proceedings published by the National Academies of Sciences, Engineering, and Medicine chronicle the presentations and discussions at a workshop, symposium, or other event convened by the National Academies. The statements and opinions contained in proceedings are those of the participants and are not endorsed by other participants, the planning committee, or the National Academies.

Rapid Expert Consultations published by the National Academies of Sciences, Engineering, and Medicine are authored by subject-matter experts on narrowly focused topics that can be supported by a body of evidence. The discussions contained in rapid expert consultations are considered those of the authors and do not contain policy recommendations. Rapid expert consultations are reviewed by the institution before release.

For information about other products and activities of the National Academies, please visit www.nationalacademies.org/about/whatwedo.

PLANNING COMMITTEE ON METHADONE TREATMENT FOR OPIOID USE DISORDER: EXAMINING FEDERAL REGULATIONS AND LAWS[1]

ALAN LESHNER (*Chair*), American Association for the Advancement of Science (Emeritus)
GAVIN BART, Hennepin County Medical Center; University of Minnesota
RICHARD BONNIE, University of Virginia
MAGDALENA CERDÁ, New York University
ABBY COULTER, Urban Survivors Union
BRIDGET DOOLING, George Washington University
SHERI DOYLE, The Pew Charitable Trusts
TRACIE GARDNER, Legal Action Center
HELENA HANSEN, University of California, Los Angeles
VAN INGRAM, Kentucky Office of Drug Control Policy
MATTHEW LAWRENCE, Emory University School of Law
GAIL MATTOX, Morehouse School of Medicine
JOSIAH "JODY" RICH, Brown University
DANIELLE RUSSELL, Sonoran Prevention Works
KENNETH STOLLER, Johns Hopkins University
JONATHAN H. WATANABE, University of California, Irvine School of Pharmacy & Pharmaceutical Sciences

Staff

CLARE STROUD, Senior Program Officer
SHEENA M. POSEY NORRIS, Program Officer
EDEN NELEMAN, Senior Program Assistant
ELIZABETH FINKELMAN, Senior Program Officer (*until December 2021*)
ALEXANDRA ANDRADA, Program Officer
AISHA SALMAN, Program Officer
NOAH DUFF, Associate Program Officer
ANDREW M. POPE, Senior Director, Board on Health Sciences Policy
SHARYL NASS, Senior Director, Board on Health Care Services

---

[1] The National Academies of Sciences, Engineering, and Medicine's planning committees are solely responsible for organizing the workshop, identifying topics, and choosing speakers. The responsibility for the published Proceedings of a Workshop rests with the workshop rapporteurs and the institution.

Reviewers

This Proceedings of a Workshop was reviewed in draft form by individuals chosen for their diverse perspectives and technical expertise. The purpose of this independent review is to provide candid and critical comments that will assist the National Academies of Sciences, Engineering, and Medicine in making each published proceedings as sound as possible and to ensure that it meets the institutional standards for quality, objectivity, evidence, and responsiveness to the charge. The review comments and draft manuscript remain confidential to protect the integrity of the process.

We thank the following individuals for their review of this proceedings:

CHINAZO CUNNINGHAM, New York State Office of Addiction Services and Supports
JASON KLETTER, BayMark Health Services
DANIEL SLEDGE, Williamson County, Texas
SCOTT STEIGER, University of California, San Francisco
SHELLY WEIZMAN, Georgetown University
DANIEL WERB, University of California, San Diego

Although the reviewers listed above provided many constructive comments and suggestions, they were not asked to endorse the content of the proceedings nor did they see the final draft before its release. The review of this proceedings was overseen by **BRIAN STROM,** Rutgers, The State

University of New Jersey. He was responsible for making certain that an independent examination of this proceedings was carried out in accordance with standards of the National Academies and that all review comments were carefully considered. Responsibility for the final content rests entirely with the rapporteurs and the National Academies.

Contents

1 INTRODUCTION AND BACKGROUND ... 1
Workshop Objectives, 3
Organization of Proceedings, 3

2 METHADONE TREATMENT: PERSONAL PERSPECTIVES ... 7
Sustained Recovery May Require Continued Methadone
 Treatment, 8
Recovery May Take Many Forms, 10
The Need for a Patient-Centered Focus, 11

3 THE HISTORY OF METHADONE AND BARRIERS TO
ACCESS FOR DIFFERENT POPULATIONS ... 13
The Early Years of Methadone Maintenance Regulation
 and the Politics of Stigma and Racialization, 15
Current Barriers to Access, Initiation, and Retention in
 Methadone Treatment, 16

4 CURRENT FEDERAL PRIORITIES AND REGULATORY
FLEXIBILITIES DURING THE COVID-19 PANDEMIC ... 29
Goals and Priorities of the Current Administration, 31
Regulatory Change in the Wake of Necessity: Lessons Learned
 from COVID-19, 38
Understanding the Disconnect between State and Federal
 Regulations, 41

5 IMPROVING ACCESS TO QUALITY TREATMENT IN OPIOID TREATMENT PROGRAMS THROUGH REGULATORY INNOVATION   45
   Federal Statutes and Regulations that Govern Opioid Treatment Programs, 47
   Pharmacy Dispensing as an Extension of OTPs, 49
   Mobile Medication Units—A Demonstration Project in New Jersey, 53
   OTPs as Hub Sites in Systemic Expansion, 54
   Other Strategies to Expand Access through OTPs Proposed by Individual Workshop Participants, 55

6 IMPROVING ACCESS TO QUALITY TREATMENT IN THE CRIMINAL JUSTICE SYSTEM AND OTHER INSTITUTIONAL SETTINGS   59
   Crosscutting Regulatory Issues that Impact Correctional Facilities and Other Institutions, 60
   Transitioning from Incarceration to the Community, 63
   A State Trial Court Perspective, 66
   Civil Rights Litigation to Enable Methadone Treatment in Institutions, 68

7 EXPANDING ACCESS TO METHADONE THROUGH REGULATORY INNOVATION: ENVISIONING APPROACHES OUTSIDE THE OPIOID TREATMENT PROGRAM SYSTEM   73
   Office-Based Methadone, 75
   International Models of Pharmacy-Based Dispensing, 77
   Innovative Models of Initiation under Existing Regulations— Inpatient and Outpatient Settings, 79
   Potential New Treatment Modalities and Settings that Could be Opened Up with Regulatory Changes, 82

8 ENSURING EQUITABLE ACCESS TO METHADONE BY REMOVING CURRENT BARRIERS AND PROVIDING INCENTIVES   89
   Regulatory Opportunities to Remove Current Barriers, 90
   Regulatory Incentives to Facilitate Access to Quality Treatment, 92

9	**FRAMEWORKS TO GUIDE THE ASSESSMENT OF LEGAL AND REGULATORY CHALLENGES**	97
	A Policy Analysis Framework to Support Health Policy Decisions, 98	
	A Cost-Effectiveness Framework to Assess Potential Legal and Regulatory Changes, 100	
10	**MOVING FORWARD: POTENTIAL CONCRETE LEGAL AND REGULATORY ACTIONS**	105
	Legal and Regulatory Reforms, 106	
	Exploring Opportunities to Reform Methadone Treatment, 109	
	Reforming Methadone Treatment within the Broader Context for Improving Access to Medications for Opioid Use Disorder, 110	
	Closing Remarks, 115	

APPENDIXES

A	REFERENCES	117
B	WORKSHOP AGENDA	125
C	COMMISSIONED PAPERS	135
	The Politics of Stigma and Racialization in the Early Years of Methadone Maintenance Regulation—*Samuel Kelton Roberts*, 136	
	Federal Administrative Pathways to Promote Access to Quality Methadone Treatment—*Matthew Lawrence*, 152	
	Innovations in Methadone Medication for Opioid Use Disorder—A Scoping Review—*Wes Williams*, 160	

1

Introduction and Background[1]

Methadone is a Food and Drug Administration– (FDA-) approved synthetic opioid agonist that is widely used for treating both pain and opioid use disorder (OUD), a chronic brain disease defined as "a problematic pattern of opioid use leading to clinically significant impairment or distress" (APA, 2022). OUD affects more than 2.7 million people in the United States aged 12 and older (APA, 2022; SAMHSA, 2021). To address barriers associated with the use of methadone to treat OUD, on March 3 and 4, 2022, the National Academies of Sciences, Engineering, and Medicine (National Academies) hosted a workshop on "Methadone Treatment for Opioid Use Disorder: Examining Federal Regulations and Laws,"[2] at the request of the Office of National Drug Control Policy (ONDCP) in the Executive Office of the President. The meeting was convened under the auspices of the National Academies boards on Health Sciences Policy and Health Care Services and the National Academy of Medicine's Action Collaborative on Countering the U.S. Opioid Epidemic.

---

[1] The planning committee's role was limited to planning the workshop, and the Proceedings of a Workshop was prepared by the workshop rapporteurs as a factual summary of what occurred at the workshop. Statements, recommendations, and opinions expressed are those of individual presenters and participants; have not been endorsed or verified by the National Academies of Sciences, Engineering, and Medicine; and should not be construed as reflecting any group consensus.

[2] To learn more about the National Academies workshop, go to https://www.nationalacademies.org/event/03-03-2022/methadone-treatment-for-opioid-use-disorder-examining-federal-regulations-and-laws-a-workshop (accessed April 26, 2022).

In his introductory remarks, Rahul Gupta, director of ONDCP, said access to methadone is hindered by many unnecessary barriers. "Methadone is often viewed in a stigmatizing way, so we need to improve both how it's viewed and how it's utilized[used] and ask the right questions that would inform our policy decisions around it," said Gupta. He noted that more than 100,000 Americans died from drug overdose in the most recent 12-month period for which data were available, and that opioids were involved in more than 78,000 of these deaths (Ahmad et al., 2021). "On average we're losing an American to an overdose every 5 minutes," he said. "These are sons and daughters, parents and grandparents, uncles and aunts, and we're losing these folks around the clock. It is heartbreaking. It is staggering. And frankly, it's unacceptable."

The workshop, chaired by Alan Leshner, chief executive officer emeritus of the American Association for the Advancement of Science and a former director of the National Institute on Drug Abuse (NIDA) of the National Institutes of Health (NIH), built on a 2019 report by the National Academies entitled *Medications for Opioid Use Disorder Save Lives* (NASEM, 2019). This report concluded that treatment of OUD with methadone, buprenorphine, or extended-release naltrexone is effective and saves lives and that long-term treatment is associated with improved outcomes, yet the report also found inequitable access to treatment across population subgroups and treatment settings.

Of the three FDA-approved drugs, methadone is the subject to the most stringent regulations, including the requirement that it is provided only through opioid treatment programs (OTPs).[3,4] Today there are about 1,900

---

[3] An OTP is a federally accredited and certified treatment program that uses medication to treat individuals with OUD. They must meet the Substance Abuse and Mental Health Services Administration's (SAMHSA's) "opioid treatment standards and the accreditation standards of SAMHSA-approved accrediting bodies," conform with federal regulations governing treatment of substance use disorders, be licensed by the state in which they operate, and be registered with the Drug Enforcement Administration. For more information, go to https://www.samhsa.gov/medication-assisted-treatment/become-accredited-opioid-treatment-program (accessed May 5, 2022).

[4] Like the other approved medications (buprenorphine and naltrexone), methadone works by targeting the mu-opioid receptor within the endogenous opioid system, but does so via a different mechanism of action and has different pharmacologic, pharmacodynamic, and pharmacokinetic properties, according to the report. Methadone is a full opioid agonist, activating opioid receptors similarly to the action of illicit opioids, while buprenorphine is a partial opioid agonist. Naltrexone is not an opioid, but a full antagonist of the mu-opioid receptor. The National Academies report concluded that while all three of these medications are effective and save lives, the most appropriate medication varies by individual and may change over time (NASEM, 2019).

OTPs in the United States,[5] with the number of OTPs expanding in the past few years despite the COVID-19 pandemic, which many policy makers predicted would result in the closure of many sites. However, despite the expansion in the number of OTPs, many individuals face substantial access barriers due to restrictive zoning ordinances, lack of third-party reimbursement, and highly regulated operating requirements at the state level, said Mark Parrino, president of the American Association for the Treatment of Opioid Dependence (AATOD). "We have to do better," said Abby Coulter, methadone liaison for Urban Survivors Union. "This workshop must be the starting point for access to methadone beyond the walls of the clinic system," she added.

Leshner predicted that the workshop would provide "landmark opportunities to seriously begin to address the longstanding issue of inadequate access to this life-saving medication…and to develop strategies to finally address a longstanding and pernicious health and social disparity."

WORKSHOP OBJECTIVES

The workshop was designed to examine the current federal regulatory and legal landscape around the provision of and access to methadone for the treatment of OUD, said Leshner (see Box 1-1). Gupta added that he hoped the workshop would explore potential policy changes to address federal, state, and local barriers to the provision of methadone treatment and consider opportunities for implementing office-based methadone treatment.

ORGANIZATION OF PROCEEDINGS

Throughout the workshop, participants examined the history and current status of methadone treatment for OUD and were asked to consider potential next steps to address regulatory and legal barriers to improve access to methadone treatment. Workshop participants explored opportunities for innovation within the current system and in settings outside OTPs. Each chapter begins with a "highlights" box that summarizes key themes and, in many cases, concludes with bulleted lists of potential policy changes and next steps proposed by individual participants. The purpose of the workshop was not to reach consensus, so many individual ideas are presented. Given the interconnectedness of the issues discussed, many of these ideas arose in different sessions of the workshop and therefore appear in multiple parts of this proceedings. Throughout this proceedings, the

---

[5] For more information, go to the Substance Abuse and Mental Health Services Administration's opioid treatment program directory available at https://dpt2.samhsa.gov/treatment (accessed June 12, 2022).

> **BOX 1-1**
> **Statement of Task**
>
> A planning committee of the National Academies of Sciences, Engineering, and Medicine will organize and conduct a 2-day public workshop that brings together experts and key stakeholders to examine the current federal regulatory and legal landscape regarding provision of and access to methadone for the treatment of opioid use disorder.
> Invited presentations and discussions will be designed to:
>
> - Examine current federal regulations governing methadone treatment services, including the current COVID-19 emergency regulatory relief;
> - Discuss the impact of these regulations relative to other factors affecting treatment services;
> - Explore potential options for modifying federal regulations and laws to expand access to quality treatment with methadone; and
> - Explore state laws that may conflict with federal regulations.
>
> The planning committee will develop the agenda for the workshop, select and invite speakers and discussants, and moderate the discussions. A proceedings of the presentations and discussions at the workshop will be prepared by a designated rapporteur in accordance with institutional guidelines.

rapporteurs aimed to use currently accepted terms that avoid perpetuating negative biases and stigma around addiction.[6] However, in some instances, presenters used other terms with a particular intention, such as to report on historical usage or the stigma they faced, and these may be reported verbatim in quotation marks.

Chapter 2 highlights three individuals' personal journeys through the methadone treatment system. A historical perspective on policies regarding methadone maintenance is presented in Chapter 3, along with discussions of how these policies create barriers to certain population groups. Chapter 4 provides an overview of the current regulatory landscape as well as flexibilities instituted in response to the COVID-19 pandemic. Improving access to treatment at OTPs through regulatory innovation is discussed in Chapter 5. Chapter 6 discusses the high prevalence of OUD in correctional facilities and opportunities for improving access to treatment at those facilities. Regulatory innovation outside of OTPs also has the potential to expand

---

[6] To learn more about terms to use and avoid when talking about addiction, go to this National Institute on Drug Abuse resource: https://nida.nih.gov/nidamed-medical-health-professionals/health-professions-education/words-matter-terms-to-use-avoid-when-talking-about-addiction (accessed June 9, 2022).

access to methadone, including among racially minoritized populations, and is discussed in Chapter 7. Chapter 8 discusses regulatory changes and incentives that could be made under current laws to help ensure equitable access to methadone. Chapter 9 presents a policy analysis framework and an economic analysis framework that could be used to inform legal and regulatory changes. Chapter 10 provides a synthesis of potential next steps proposed by individual workshop participants to improve access to quality methadone treatment. References cited throughout these proceedings are listed in Appendix A, the workshop agenda is in Appendix B, and three commissioned papers serving as background to the workshop are provided in Appendix C.

2

Methadone Treatment: Personal Perspectives

HIGHLIGHTS

- Opioid use disorder (OUD) is a chronic brain disorder, not a consequence of bad behavior (Ginter).
- Patients receiving medications for opioid use disorder (MOUD) deserve to be treated with dignity and respect, but often face stigma and prejudice (B. Davis).
- Treatment for OUD is more than just medication. Supports designed specifically for individual needs of people on methadone are essential to facilitate recovery (B. Davis, Ginter).
- Practitioners who provide MOUD should be trained in methadone pharmacology and should understand how a patient's needs may change during different stages of recovery (B. Davis).
- The complex biopsychosocial nature of OUD may require, in addition to medication, comprehensive services to address trauma and other diseases such as hepatitis C and HIV (B. Davis).
- Some patients may need to take an opioid agonist to feel well and function normally (Coulter).
- Policy changes that could improve MOUD include providing access to methadone beyond clinic walls and aligning federal and state regulations (Coulter).

- Denying take-homes doses and forcing patients to undergo counseling because of a positive opioid screen may reverse progress that has been made in recovery (Coulter).
- It is important not to discount the positive outcomes patients might experience at an opioid treatment program through its integrated care model (B. Davis).

NOTE: This list is the rapporteurs' summary of points made by the individual speakers identified, and the statements have not been endorsed or verified by the National Academies of Sciences, Engineering, and Medicine. They are not intended to reflect a consensus among workshop participants.

To infuse discussions pertaining to potential policy changes with a better understanding of the needs of individuals with lived experience, the workshop opened with three individuals' personal journeys and their reflections on the benefits of methadone treatment, challenges they have encountered related to the provision and access to treatment, and considerations on how best to move forward. It is important to recognize that the experiences of individuals who take methadone for OUD are as varied and diverse as the people themselves; these three perspectives are meant to illustrate personal experiences but cannot fully represent the broad array of experiences or people who have been affected by the current regulatory and legal landscape regulating to how methadone is dispensed and administered.

SUSTAINED RECOVERY MAY REQUIRE CONTINUED METHADONE TREATMENT

Walter Ginter, project director of the Medication-Assisted Recovery Support (MARS™) Project, introduced himself as a person in sustained methadone-assisted recovery from heroin. In 1972, after only 2 years serving in the U.S. Army, Ginter was discharged for being a heroin user. In 1977, he began methadone treatment for the first time.

Shortly after beginning treatment, Ginter stopped using heroin, got married, and had a good job. "I could have been a poster child for methadone treatment," he said. When a new job opportunity became available, his boss told him, "First, I want you to get off that 'junkie drug,'[1] methadone."

---

[1] As noted in Chapter 1, in some instances throughout this proceedings, the rapporteurs deviated from currently accepted terms when necessary to capture the language used by a speaker when they selected it to make a certain point about the stigma they faced.

Ginter successfully completed a 30-day detox program, but had a recurrence of heroin use just 3 days later.

Ginter started methadone treatment again, and "after a few years, again [he] was doing very well." He and his wife had started a business and were doing well. A counselor in the program suggested he might want to taper off methadone, but he relapsed again when he got to about 5 milligrams. This pattern repeated itself over the next 20 years as Ginter went in and out of at least eight methadone programs.

"I finally realized there must be more to this treatment than just the medication," he said. A psychologist assigned to him by the Fairfield County, CT, Alcohol and Drug Prevention Council offered him the opportunity to beat up a 6-foot teddy bear with a baseball bat. "I tried to explain to her that I had addiction issues, not anger issues, but she didn't seem to understand the difference," said Ginter. This experience taught him several valuable lessons: First, being smart and financially stable did not lead to successful recovery, but, equally as important, the supports provided need to be specifically designed for methadone patients.

Ginter began to believe that his inability to get off methadone reflected some sort of innate weakness. Then, a website he created for methadone patients came to the attention of Joyce Woods, who was then president of the National Alliance on Medication Assisted Recovery (NAMA Recovery). Woods explained to Ginter that he had a chronic brain disorder. Ginter said it was the first time in 20 years of treatment that anyone told him opioid addiction was not due to bad behavior but to a brain disorder. "She said, 'You may be on methadone for the rest of your life, but what difference does it make? Your life is everything you want it to be.'" Ginter started working with NAMA Recovery as an advocate with the goal of sharing this revelation with others. With colleagues, he wrote and received funding for a grant from the Substance Abuse and Mental Health Services Administration (SAMHSA) to establish the MARS Project,[2] the first project ever funded to provide recovery support services for people on methadone. At the Albert Einstein College of Medicine, he started training others about implementing medication and recovery services and was awarded another SAMHSA grant to establish the MARS Training Institute. Since then, Ginter said he has done training in 31 states and made 5 trips to Vietnam, which now offers MARS services nationwide.

The saying "timing is everything" held true for Ginter, who notes that if he were trying to set up a program in another country or even go to another state to train today, his methadone maintenance program would require him to seek approval to leave the state. "You can't understand how

---

[2] For more information about the MARS™ Project, go to https://marsproject.org (accessed May 5, 2022).

demeaning it is for someone on medical maintenance for 21 years to suddenly be treated just like a junkie," he said. "If I was on buprenorphine and could see a private doctor under similar terms as medical maintenance, it would be a much better situation."

RECOVERY MAY TAKE MANY FORMS

In recovery for nearly 30 years, Brenda Davis works as a patient advocate with NAMA Recovery. Like Ginter and many others, recovery was a process. It started when, under the influence of pills and heroin, she had a massive seizure in front of her young daughter. Only a few weeks earlier, her little girl had watched as Davis and a friend were up for days using drugs. Davis finally fell asleep, waking up around 24 hours later to a baby banging her in the head with a bottle because she was hungry. "She'd cried so long that she just didn't have any more tears," said Davis. "Although I felt bad about it, I couldn't stop at the time. But the seizure was the one thing that changed my life. I saw the hurt in my baby's face and knew that was my bottom."

Davis entered a methadone treatment program that provided her the structure and support she needed. At first, she said she wasn't ready to be in control of her own medication. "My first thought was that if I got weekend bottles, I could split one to get myself through the weekend and sell the other," she recalled. "If I didn't have the structure of the program, I don't think the outcome would have been the same."

Eventually, Davis said she was able to "literally, emotionally, and psychologically move forward" and became solid in her recovery. She started a career in treatment, became manager of a clinic, and then took on a patient advocacy role in a large hospital. She got her bachelor's degree and went on to earn a master's degree in social work. After working in the opioid treatment field for more than 25 years, she said she believes she has found her true calling.

Part of her job, she said, is to "help patients understand the true meaning of recovery," and to imbue in patients the conviction that they should be treated with dignity and respect. "I look through the lens of a patient, but also a woman of color," she said. "I know what it's like to not be treated as a person, and I understand the struggles we continue to face in medication-assisted treatment due to stigma and prejudice."

Davis is also a strong advocate for patients having access to practitioners who understand OUD and are trained in methadone pharmacology. "History has shown us what happens when untrained practitioners prescribe methadone. The ultimate patient harm, death, often occurs," she said. At the same time, patients require access to trained professionals who understand the differing needs of patients at different stages of their recovery. Indeed, she said, data show that integrated care offered through opioid treatment programs (OTPs) results in positive long-term outcomes for many patients. However, stable patients who no longer need or want counseling, case management, and other wraparound services deserve the option of moving to office-based methadone treatment and/or new models of pharmacy-based prescribing.

She added that the complex biopsychosocial[3] nature of OUD means that treatment requires more than access to medication. Methadone does not treat trauma, hepatitis C, or HIV, she said. "Patients deserve to have comprehensive services, but we also deserve not to be forced into boxes that we do not need or want."

This point is explored further in Chapter 10 in terms of redefining "success" in methadone treatment to include non-abstinence-based recovery.

THE NEED FOR A PATIENT-CENTERED FOCUS

Abby Coulter introduced herself as "a photographer, a parent, a daughter, a friend, an activist, and a person on methadone." She is also a coauthor of the *Methadone Manifesto*,[4] a document that outlines many policy issues related to methadone treatment and proposes a vision for change from the lens of people with lived experience. Her journey began nearly 20 years ago when she walked into a methadone clinic as a pregnant woman on drugs. The clinic system that existed at that time was welcoming, helpful, and patient centered, said Coulter, in stark contrast to what exists today.

Coulter came to understand that she was a person who needs to take an opioid agonist to feel well. She spent the next 19 years trying to navigate a system that, she said, "has increasingly failed to focus on evidence-based, patient-centered care." Then, despite 20 years of being a successful, compliant methadone patient, she had a positive screen for an opioid and lost everything. Denied access to take-home medication, she was forced to go into the clinic for daily dosing and start inpatient counseling. "The idea that all of the work I had put in was stripped away in the blink of an eye, without a single thought of how that was going to affect everything I had

---

[3] Biopsychosocial is defined as "relating to, or concerned with the biological, psychological, and social aspects in contrast to the strictly biomedical aspects of disease" according to the Merriam-Webster Dictionary; https://www.merriam-webster.com/medical/biopsychosocial (accessed June 8, 2022).

[4] To learn more about the *Methadone Manifesto*, go to https://sway.office.com/UjvQx4Z NnXAYxhe7?ref=Link (accessed May 9, 2022).

worked for, was a terrible feeling," she said. The clinic system and methadone maintenance should not get in the way of progress, said Coulter, yet that was exactly what happened to her.

"We have to do better," said Coulter. She advocated for access to methadone beyond the clinic walls and alignment of federal and state regulations. She did note that during the COVID-19 pandemic, SAMHSA modified some regulations. "It took a pandemic, an overdose crisis of epic tragic loss, and a failed war on drugs to recognize that what has existed for far too long isn't working anymore."

3

The History of Methadone and Barriers to Access for Different Populations

HIGHLIGHTS

- Methadone is not only one of the most closely regulated medical treatments, but also one of the most stigmatized, controversial, and misunderstood (Roberts).
- Though used as an analgesic since the 1930s, methadone emerged as a narcotics maintenance treatment modality for heroin dependence in the 1960s, and by 1972, following a regulatory history derived from the politics of stigma and distrust, the U.S. Food and Drug Administration and Bureau of Narcotics instituted stringent access restrictions (Roberts).
- Opioid overdose death rates have skyrocketed in the past 20 years, with the greatest increases in Black Americans (Cerdá).
- Increased access to medications for opioid use disorder has the power to substantially reduce overdose rates (Cerdá).
- In comparison to buprenorphine, which can be prescribed by a health care provider with prescribing privileges and dispensed at a pharmacy, methadone must be obtained at an opioid treatment program, often requiring patients to travel long distances and wait in line (Cerdá).
- Social barriers to methadone access include affordability, stigma, discrimination in health care settings, lack of culturally responsive care, and inequalities in the criminal justice system (Cerdá).

- Pregnancy is a critical moment for treating opioid use disorder (OUD) given the near-universal health insurance for pregnant people and their motivation to protect their unborn child; however, because of physiological changes during pregnancy, once-daily dosing, required by federal statutes, is often insufficient (Terplan).
- Treatment attrition caused by a lack of, or non-continuation of health insurance or Medicare is associated with increased maternal deaths, particularly in the postpartum period (Terplan).
- Punitive state policies regarding substance use and pregnancy contribute to worse obstetric outcomes (Terplan).
- Substance use is a primary driver of increased foster care placements, which in combination with racial inequities, create a child welfare system that often leads to parental custody termination (Terplan).
- The unique health inequities faced by LGBTQIA+ individuals and those living with HIV include disparities in the treatment for OUD and must be understood in the context of a minority stress framework (Keuroghlian).
- Medication as well as behavioral health approaches, delivered in a culturally responsive way, are needed to treat OUD in LGBTQIA+ individuals (Keuroghlian).
- Older adults are at increased risk for chronic pain conditions and metabolize methadone differently, but regulations require patients to be free of illicit drug use in order to receive take-home doses, limiting the ability for older adults to receive appropriate methadone treatment for OUD (Levander).
- Co-occurring conditions in older adults that limit mobility and cognition can make receiving methadone prohibitively challenging (Levander).

NOTE: This list is the rapporteurs' summary of points made by the individual speakers identified, and the statements have not been endorsed or verified by the National Academies of Sciences, Engineering, and Medicine. They are not intended to reflect a consensus among workshop participants.

"Our methadone system is unique to the U.S. and evolved through the accident of our history and politics," said Helena Hansen, professor of psychiatry and chair of the research theme in translational social science and health equity at the University of California at Los Angeles David Geffen School of Medicine, and moderator of the first workshop session. Moreover, she said, "Understanding how that happened helps us to see that our current regulations could be otherwise."

THE EARLY YEARS OF METHADONE MAINTENANCE REGULATION AND THE POLITICS OF STIGMA AND RACIALIZATION

According to Samuel Kelton Roberts, associate professor of history, sociomedical sciences, and African American and African diaspora studies at Columbia University, methadone maintenance[1] is one of the most closely regulated medical protocols. "Perhaps not entirely by coincidence, it is also one of the most stigmatized, controversial, and misunderstood," he said. Stigma alienates patients from treatments such as methadone maintenance, said Roberts. Black patients are particularly affected by a trifecta of stigmas—being Black, having an opioid use disorder, and being a methadone patient—which, combined with the history of medical abuses against people of color, has engendered a culture of mistrust, he said. Roberts' ideas are further developed in the commissioned paper that can be found in Appendix C.

Methadone emerged as a maintenance treatment modality for heroin dependence in the mid-1960s. Mark Parrino, added that opioid treatment programs (OTPs) came into existence because of a rejection by the medical community to treat this particular patient population.

By 1972, the Food and Drug Administration (FDA) and the Drug Enforcement Administration (DEA) had instituted severe regulations that restricted access, said Roberts. These regulations were designed primarily to prevent methadone from being diverted to the street, he said. For example, patients were required to receive medication under close supervision at federally approved clinics and submit to regular urine testing. Some states also employed coercive tactics, such as requiring participation in a methadone program in order to receive public benefits or to obtain release from prison, said Roberts. Physicians were also subject to close scrutiny and were required to have complicated security systems to prevent diversion.

"When the FDA created this restrictive environment and Congress bifurcated authority between DEA and what would ultimately be SAMHSA,"

---

[1] Methadone maintenance treatment was the term used most frequently in the historical period discussed here. The preferred term today is medication for opioid use disorder (MOUD).

recalled Parrino, "I will tell you without any reservation that it was sort of akin to the Wild West prior to the implementation of the regulations."

Roberts said policies instituted at that time affect how methadone treatment is viewed. When a treatment is heavily regulated, he said, people assume that it is dangerous. Another common criticism of methadone is that it is portrayed as a "false cure," merely substituting one drug for another, said Roberts.

Public mistrust of methadone as a useful medical intervention increased when many politicians began promoting it more for its ability to reduce crime than for its therapeutic potential, said Roberts. Regulations were also instituted against a backdrop of increasing calls from Black grassroots organizations for community involvement in policy decisions relevant to the Black community. Yet, local community health and antipoverty organizations were excluded from policy discussions, increasing the alienation of those communities and contributing to the perception that methadone could be weaponized as an agent of social control and even genocide, said Roberts.

CURRENT BARRIERS TO ACCESS, INITIATION, AND RETENTION IN METHADONE TREATMENT

With an understanding of the historical backdrop to methadone regulations in the United States, several workshop participants discussed the effects of those regulations on health inequities, including social barriers to treatment, and considerations for special populations. Those populations include minoritized groups; people with low income; elderly individuals; people involved in the criminal justice system; pregnant women; lesbian, gay, bisexual, transgender, queer, intersex, asexual and all sexual and gender minority (LGBTQIA+) individuals; and individuals with HIV/AIDS.

Racial and Ethnic Minorities: High Risks, High Barriers

Opioid overdose death rates have skyrocketed in the past 20 years in all racial and ethnic groups, with the greatest increase among Black Americans in the past 10 years, said Magdalena Cerdá, professor and director of the Center for Opioid Epidemiology and Policy at the Department of Population Health, New York University Grossman School of Medicine (Friedman et al., 2022). The COVID-19 pandemic has exacerbated the crisis further, she said. In 2021, more than 100,000 people died from opioid overdoses, with particularly high increases among racially minoritized groups, especially Black Americans, followed by people of Asian and Hispanic ancestry (Baumgartner and Radley, 2022) (see Figure 3-1).

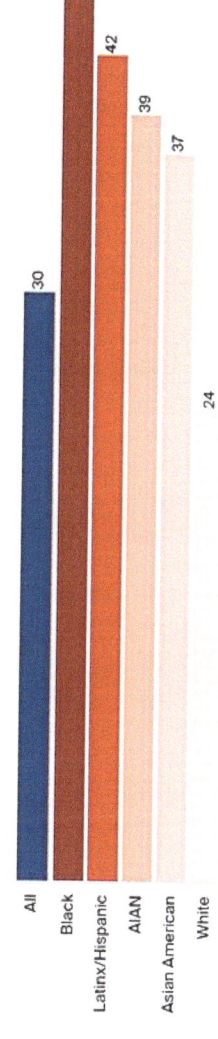

FIGURE 3-1 Opioid overdose death rates by race/ethnicity January–December 2020 versus January–December 2019. All demographic groups experienced more overdose deaths during 2020, with the steepest rise among Black Americans.
NOTE: AIAN = American Indian/Alaska Native.
SOURCES: Presented by Magdalena Cerdá, March 3, 2022; Baumgartner and Radley, 2022; CDC, 2021.

Cerdá noted that studies have shown that increased access to medications for opioid use disorder (MOUD) has the power to substantially reduce overdose rates. "What is particularly tragic is that racially minoritized individuals, who are experiencing some of the greatest rises in overdose rates today, have less access to medications for opioid use disorder," said Cerdá.

In a study comparing the number of people who meet the criteria for OUD with those who actually receive treatment, Cerdá and colleagues documented a huge gap, as well as disparities in who gets access to treatment (this study is under review). Other studies have shown similar inequities across racial lines, said Cerdá (Wu et al., 2016). Indeed, one study showed that White patients are more likely to be referred to a medical professional and receive medication as part of their treatment plan, and less likely to leave against medical advice or be terminated by the facility than are racially minoritized patients (Entress, 2021). Regions with large Black and Hispanic populations have also been shown to have reduced access to hospitals that offer medication-based treatment (Chang et al., 2022).

Looking specifically at access to methadone and buprenorphine, Cerdá noted additional examples of racial patterning, with racially minoritized individuals having lower access to buprenorphine, which she called a "more flexible form of care" (Schiff et al., 2020). Whereas buprenorphine can be accessed through a primary care provider or psychiatrist with a prescription that can be picked up at a pharmacy and consumed in the comfort of their own home, access to methadone is much more difficult, said Cerdá. Access to methadone requires people to attend a licensed OTP as often as 6 days per week, said Cerdá. They sometimes must stand in line outside waiting for treatment. "This is in itself a highly stigmatized, punitive approach to getting access to treatment," said Cerdá.

Geographical differences in access to buprenorphine and methadone treatment also contribute to racial patterning, said Cerdá. A study in New York City by Helena Hansen and colleagues showed that between 2004 and 2013, buprenorphine treatment increased across all areas, with a significantly higher increase in areas with the highest income and lowest percentage of Black, Hispanic, and lower income residents. By contrast, methadone use was concentrated in areas of high poverty and a higher concentration of Black and Hispanic residents, said Cerdá (Hansen et al., 2016). Cerdá and colleagues observed a similar pattern when they analyzed data from more than 3,000 counties across the United States. Methadone was more likely to be available in counties with highly segregated Black populations, whereas buprenorphine was more likely to be available in highly segregated White communities (Goedel et al., 2020).

Cerdá suggested that to reduce racial and ethnic inequalities in access to MOUD, regulatory and social barriers need to be dismantled. The first regulatory barrier she cited is the restriction of methadone to specialized licensed programs. This limits access because people are often required to travel far from home to get treatment. She noted that this is a particularly acute problem for rural populations. Second, Cerdá said, requiring people to attend a facility to access care can be challenging for low-income people in particular, who must balance this requirement against the realities of childcare and non-flexible jobs. Requiring facilities to provide counseling presents another regulatory barrier because it makes it difficult to fully staff opioid treatment programs, resulting in a limited number of facilities licensed to provide methadone, Cerdá added.

Social barriers include affordability (including the cost of copays), insurance and Medicaid-imposed limits on the duration and dose of treatment for methadone, and prior authorization requirements, said Cerdá. Beyond these factors related to the cost of treatment, other social barriers to methadone treatment include stigma, discrimination in health care settings, lack of culturally responsive and respectful care, and the inequalities present in the criminal justice system. "We know that there are racial and ethnic inequalities in arrests and incarceration," said Cerdá. "At the same time, we know that for every day spent incarcerated, the likelihood of initiating and being retained in treatment decreases substantially."

Cerdá suggested policy solutions that could reduce racial and ethnic inequalities in access to MOUD. She cited a study showing that after the implementation of the Affordable Care Act, Black patients were more likely to access MOUD, particularly in states that expanded Medicaid coverage. Other policies that could broaden access to MOUD include integrating methadone into office-based treatment,[2] particularly in primary care, and allowing for telehealth prescribing and pharmacy dispensing of methadone, said Cerdá. She noted that during the COVID-19 pandemic, telehealth prescribing and pharmacy dispensing were allowed for buprenorphine. The Opioid Treatment Access Act of 2022 (HR 6279[3] and S 3629[4]), introduced in the U.S. Senate by Edward Markey (D-MA) and Rand Paul (R-KY), and in the U.S. House of Representatives by Donald Norcross (D-NJ) and David Trone (D-MD), would help to achieve these goals.

Finally, Cerdá suggesting making permanent the federal requirement that Medicaid cover all medications for OUD; enacting policies to reduce copays and prior authorization requirements by commercial insurance; and expanding the possibility of using community settings to dispense methadone, including mobile units and harm reduction programs.

---

[2] Outpatient treatment services provided outside of licensed OTPs by primary care or general health prescribers with a Drug Addiction Treatment Act (DATA) waiver.

[3] To learn more about HR 6279, the Opioid Treatment Access Act of 2022, go to https://www.congress.gov/bill/117th-congress/house-bill/6279/text (accessed May 2, 2022).

[4] To learn more about S 3629, the Opioid Treatment Access Act of 2022, go to https://www.govinfo.gov/app/details/BILLS-117s3629is (accessed May 2, 2022).

Pregnancy and Parenting: A Critical Time for People with OUD

Pregnancy is a critical moment for addressing OUD because there is near-universal health insurance for pregnant people and motivation to protect their baby-to-be, said Mishka Terplan, medical director at Friends Research Institute and adjunct faculty at the University of California, San Francisco. He added that methadone and buprenorphine are the safest and most effective medications for OUD during pregnancy and improve outcomes.

However, for people with OUD, "we oftentimes abandon support during pregnancy, in particular postpartum," said Terplan. He maintained that this distinction results from a federal statute that is misaligned with the normal physiology of pregnancy, the realities of the postpartum period, and the right and dignity of parenting. He explained that during pregnancy, as the metabolism of most people shifts toward rapid or ultrarapid metabolism, increasing methadone doses may be needed, particularly later in gestation. Once-daily dosing and restrictions against take-home doses, which could enable patients to split doses over the day, may lead to overmedication following dosing and undermedication the rest of the day, he said.

Terplan also linked treatment attrition caused by the lack of or noncontinuation of health insurance or Medicare to the marked increase in maternal deaths in the United States. "Overdose is one of the leading causes of maternal death in the United States, and most of these deaths happen in the postpartum period," he said. Some of this increase in overdose deaths postpartum is due to treatment attrition, which in the case of methadone may result from discontinuation of health insurance or Medicaid after giving birth, said Terplan. Standard prenatal care also often ignores the "fourth trimester," that is, the 1-year postpartum period, he said.

Finally, he cited the proliferation of punitive state policies related to substance use in pregnancy as a driver of worse obstetric outcomes, higher rates of neonatal abstinence syndrome, and low birthweight and preterm delivery. These punitive policies are due to an increase in restrictive reproductive health policies at the state level, he said. For example, states that have restricted abortion access are more likely to collapse substance use in pregnancy with child abuse, even though he said the assumption that OUD or using drugs during pregnancy is associated with abuse or neglect is not supported by the literature. These same states are also more likely to arrest, prosecute, and convict pregnant people who miscarry while using drugs or give birth to an infant who develops symptoms of withdrawal to opioids.

Substance use is also the primary driver of increased foster care placements in the United States, added Terplan, noting that there are marked racial inequities in the child welfare system, driven in large part by primary health care providers. Terplan's research has shown that the rate of screened-in reports[5] from medical professionals has increased markedly over the past decade, particularly for Black infants, followed by Alaska Natives and American Indian infants and other minoritized populations. "The child welfare system on the whole is a system of surveillance, not of support," said Terplan.

Yet, he maintained that while a huge amount is known about early childhood development and how to support children in their development, the child welfare system and foster placement in particular interfere with that greatly. Instead of focusing on drugs and whether someone has a positive drug test, he suggested the need to "flip the script, to acknowledge what we all agree upon, which is that all children should be raised in stable communities devoid of violence so that they can thrive and reach their full potential." Until the focus is changed from drug enforcement to early childhood development, some form of discrimination and stigma is going to be inherent," said Terplan.

He advocated loosening OTP regulations to address the needs of pregnant and parenting people. Split dosing (i.e., dividing a prescribed daily dose of methadone into two or more administrations in the course of one day) is just one example of how regulatory change could result in better pregnancy outcomes. More generally, Terplan supported efforts to provide integrated child and family friendly reproductive health services at treatment sites.

At the federal level, he noted that the Child Abuse Prevention and Treatment Act (CAPTA)[6] is currently undergoing reauthorization, providing an opportunity for states to decouple substance use disorder from child abuse; to roll back punitive policies; and to implement legislation grounded in basic bioethical principles.

Unique Barriers for LGBTQIA+ Individuals and People Living with HIV

LGBTQIA+ individuals, including or as well as those living with HIV, comprise communities with unique health disparities and inequities, including in the realm of substance use disorders, said Alex Keuroghlian, associate professor of psychiatry at Harvard Medical School and director of the Division of Education and Training at The Fenway Institute. Fenway Health was founded more than 50 years ago as a historically LGBTQIA+-focused health center, said Keuroghlian. The National LGBTQIA+ Health

---

[5] A "screened-in report" is a report to state child protection agencies that will be followed up with an investigation.
[6] To learn more about CAPTA, go to www.acf.hhs.gov/cb/law-regulation/child-abuse-prevention-and-treatment-act-capta (accessed March 28, 2022).

Education Center at the Fenway Institute[7] offers educational programs, resources and consultation to health care organizations, he said. Among these resources are best practice guidelines for addressing opioid use disorders among LGBTQIA+ people.[8]

Keuroghlian cited several examples of the impact of the opioid epidemic on this population:

- Data from SAMHSA indicate that there is a higher incidence of prescription pain medication misuse among sexual minority people, and research also shows that sexual minority youth misuse prescription pain medication earlier in life than do their sexual majority counterparts, said Keuroghlian (Kecojevic et al., 2012).
- Men who have sex with men (MSM) also have higher perceived stress levels associated with higher opioid misuse (Kecojevic et al., 2015), and non-medical opioid use among MSM is associated with risky behaviors such as condomless sexual intercourse and sharing of syringes (Zule et al., 2016).
- Transgender and gender-diverse middle and high school students report increased use of prescription pain medication compared with cisgender teens, and adults on Medicare report increased levels of chronic pain, which puts them at higher risk for opioid use disorder, said Keuroghlian. In addition, when transgender and gender-diverse individuals pursue gender-affirming surgery, they are often prescribed opioids to manage their pain.
- Keuroghlian and colleagues have also shown that among transgender and gender-diverse adults, the increased prevalence of substance use is associated with intimate partner violence, posttraumatic stress disorder (PTSD), public accommodations discrimination, unstable housing, and sex work; all are viewed as downstream effects of chronic gender minority stress (Keuroghlian et al., 2015).

"This is an oppressed minoritized population with a massive built-in exposure to opioids," said Keuroghlian. "We're increasingly having conversations with public health officials and policy makers to try to mitigate the adverse public health impact of exposure."

Keuroghlian said the health inequities experienced by LGBTQIA+ people must be understood in the context of a minority stress framework. From

---

[7] To learn more about the National LGBTQIA+ Health Education Center, go to https://www.lgbtqiahealtheducation.org (accessed March 24, 2022).

[8] The publication "Addressing Opioid Use Disorder among LGBTQ Populations" is available for download at https://www.lgbtqiahealtheducation.org/publication/addressing-opioid-use-disorder-among-lgbtq-populations.

early childhood through adolescence and adulthood, LGBTQIA+ individuals experience a high level of external stigma-related stress in the form of everyday discrimination, victimization, microaggressions, and outright violence, said Keuroghlian. He noted that there is also an intersectional component to this stigma-related stress. For example, he said the Federal Bureau of Investigation has reported that African American transgender women have among the highest incidence of hate crimes in the United States.

For many people, this external stigma-related stress may lead to disruptions in psychological processes, coping skills, emotional regulation, interpersonal functioning, and protective cognitive structures and beliefs. These disruptions, combined with medical mistrust due to the historical mistreatment of LGBTQIA+ individuals in health care systems, may result in distressing beliefs, such as that their lives will never improve, or that no one can be trusted. External stigma-related stress combined with similar internal stress, such as internalized homophobia or transphobia, may also lead to an increased prevalence of behavioral health problems and depression, anxiety, PTSD, and substance use disorders, said Keuroghlian. These stressors, in turn, can lead to decreased engagement in health care, resulting in physical health problems.

Keuroghlian and colleagues have used this minority stress framework to understand the evidence on opioid use and misuse among LGBTQIA+ people and suggest behavioral health interventions using a trauma-informed approach (Girouard et al., 2019). He added that while minority stress can present as a crisis, it can also provide an opportunity to cultivate resilience and learn adaptive coping skills. However, Keuroghlian emphasized that addressing OUD in this population will require not just cultivating resilience, but more importantly, making policy and structural changes.

For example, MOUD is an important tool for treating opioid use disorders in LGBTQIA+ people, but it is not sufficient, said Keuroghlian. He advocated incorporating behavioral health approaches such as cognitive behavioral therapy, delivered in a culturally responsive manner grounded in the minority stress framework and tailored for LGBTQIA+ people. Such care would focus on minority stress-specific triggers for cravings, such as identity-related discrimination and victimization, expectations of rejection, identity concealment, and internalized homophobia/transphobia (Girouard et al., 2019).

Framing substance use disorders as barriers to personal health goals may also be useful. For example, Keuroghlian said he has found that the most compelling reason people give for maintaining abstinence from opioids is that they want to pursue gender-affirming surgery and know the surgeon would require this in order to perform the procedure with good surgical outcomes. In addition, culturally responsive biobehavioral approaches for transgender people should address medically unmonitored hormone use, particularly in Black, Indigenous, and People of Color, who often have less access to gender-affirming medical care.

Keuroghlian emphasized the importance of delivering methadone-related care in environments that are inclusive, affirming, and welcoming to the identities of LGBTQIA+ peoples (Goldhammer et al., 2021). Progress has been made in this regard through the use of electronic health records, he said. Since 2016, the Bureau of Primary Healthcare[9] has required all Federally Qualified Health Centers (FQHCs), nearly 1,400,[10] to report sexual orientation and gender identity data (Keuroghlian, 2021). "This allows us to engage in population health management and also improves culturally responsive addiction care at health centers nationally," he said, noting that more standardized data collection across health systems could improve this even further. He added that city-level non-discrimination policies related to sexual orientation and gender identity increase the completeness of reported data (Almazan et al., 2021). "So there's a real relationship between non-discrimination laws and collection of this important demographic data to be able to provide culturally responsive tailored care," said Keuroghlian.

Keuroghlian noted that many of the challenges discussed in providing methadone care to LGBTQIA+ people also extend to people living with HIV. He and his colleagues have implemented clinic-based and mobile buprenorphine interventions for this population in recent years. A similar implementation science approach is needed to evaluate and scale up such interventions in the methadone space.

Challenges for Older Adults with OUD

Current policies regarding dosing, take-homes, and where methadone can be dispensed also fail older adults with OUD, said Ximena Levander, assistant professor of medicine and clinical investigator at Oregon Health & Science University. She gave two examples, which highlight the challenges faced by older adults.

In the first example, a 60-year-old man being treated with methadone for chronic severe pain had turned to heroin when the primary care clinic where he had been treated closed and he was unable to find another clinic where he could receive methadone treatment. Levander saw him at an OTP after he had developed a severe OUD. He asked not to exceed 60 milligrams of methadone once per day because he experienced sedation at higher doses that limited his ability to function normally. However, at night when the

---

[9] To learn more about the Bureau of Primary Healthcare, go to https://bphc.hrsa.gov (accessed March 27, 2022).

[10] For more information about Federally Qualified Health Centers, go to https://bphc.hrsa.gov/about-health-centers (accessed June 14, 2022).

morning methadone dose wore off, he continued to use heroin. This led to a positive urine drug test for opioids and ineligibility for take-home doses.

Older adults are at increased risk of having musculoskeletal pain as well as co-occurring conditions that limit their ability to safely receive methadone treatment under current guidelines or those that make receiving methadone treatment prohibitively challenging, said Levander. For example, these co-occurring conditions may result in reduced mobility or cognitive impairment, making it difficult to get to an appointment even if they remember it, she said. Each co-occurring condition also increases the risk of polypharmacy, said Levander, noting that there is an extensive list of medications that interact with methadone. Moreover, the metabolism of methadone changes significantly with age. The result, she said, is that chronic pain may be better treated with methadone dosed two or three times per day depending on how it is metabolized and how it works on opioid receptors. Side effects from methadone treatment that may also be a significant concern in older adults include heart arrhythmias, respiratory depression, worsening constipation, urinary retention, and sedation, often increasing their risk for falls and injury.

Physical limitations and access challenges were a particular problem for the second patient Levander described. She was a frail 58-year-old woman with multiple medical conditions including severe opioid use disorder, which was being treated at an OTP with 80 milligrams of methadone per day. She was hospitalized with a severe heart infection called endocarditis, which caused a blood clot that caused a spinal infarct and bilateral paralysis in her legs. Her doctors recommended discharge to a skilled nursing facility (SNF), but no such facility was found that could dispense her methadone. To facilitate discharge to the SNF, there was an attempt to switch her to buprenorphine, which she was unable to tolerate. Levander recalled, "Given no options for rehabilitation, she was transitioned to comfort care and eventually died in the hospital on methadone."

This patient highlights the devastation that can result from barriers to treatment in a SNF faced by patients on methadone, said Levander. Indeed, she said, a research study found that many nursing facilities violate Americans with Disabilities Act (ADA) laws by rejecting patients for post-acute facility placement (Kimmel et al., 2021). This is discussed further in Chapter 6.

Levander mentioned several policy changes that could have prevented the tragic outcome this woman experienced. For example, while current policies require daily dosing regardless of a person's living situation, the controlled environment of a SNF could have been able to accommodate split dosing at more appropriate levels.

Other system gaps and potential policy changes discussed by Levander and other individual participants in this workshop session are summarized in Box 3-1. These include changes to Medicare reimbursement guidelines. Levander said Medicare historically did not cover treatment in an OTP, requiring patients to self-pay if they wanted to stay on methadone or if unable to pay, to transition off methadone. The Substance Use-Disorder Prevention that Promotes Opioid Recovery and Treatment for Patients and Communities (SUPPORT) Act of 2018[11] expanded addiction treatment coverage for Medicare and Medicaid. In addition, Medicare Managed Care and Advantage Plans as well as private insurance may limit coverage through requirements for cost sharing and prior authorizations. Levander advocated including methadone as a preferred drug by Medicare Part D to promote reforms such as providing methadone through pharmacies, doctors' offices, and hospitals for older adults.

Training in addiction treatment across all population groups is also critical, said Levander. "Our patients deserve to be treated by people who are trained to provide them with the best evidence-based care in a non-stigmatizing and compassionate way," she said. Keuroghlian echoed that point, noting the need for medical education reform and integration of addiction medicine into the standard curriculum at schools of medicine, nursing, and social work. He suggested that this is already happening in schools across the country, as medical educators have become more cognizant of social determinants of health and equity.

---

[11] To learn more about the SUPPORT Act and other federal regulations that pertain to medication-assisted treatment for OTPs, go to https://www.samhsa.gov/medication-assisted-treatment/statutes-regulations-guidelines (accessed April 6, 2022).

BOX 3-1
Potential Policy Ideas Proposed by Individual Workshop Participants to Address Inequities in Methadone Access

- Expanding Medicaid coverage (Cerdá).
- Expanding the availability of methadone in community settings, including primary care practices, mobile vans, and harm reduction facilities (Cerdá, Keuroghlian).
- Allowing telehealth prescribing and pharmacy dispensing of methadone (Cerdá).
- Requiring Medicaid to cover all medications for opioid use disorder (Cerdá).
- Enacting policies to reduce copays and prior authorization requirements (Cerdá).
- Modifying opioid treatment program (OTP) regulations to address needs of pregnant and parenting people, for example, allowing split dosing for this population group (Terplan).
- Enacting policies that provide integrated child and family-friendly reproductive services at OTPs (Terplan).
- Decoupling substance use from child abuse, roll back punitive policies, and ensure legislation reflects basic bioethical principles during the reauthorization of the Child Abuse Prevention and Treatment Act (Terplan).
- Revising Medicare reimbursement guidelines for methadone, including requirements for cost sharing and prior authorizations (Levander).
- Instituting value-based payment models for methadone coverage and develop mechanisms for aligning reimbursement with evidence-based care (Levander, Terplan).
- Requiring that methadone be included as a preferred drug by Medicare Part D providers, and require skilled nursing facilities to provide methadone to patients treated for opioid use disorder (Levander).
- Reforming medical education to integrate addiction medicine and courses on social determinants of health and equity into the curricula at schools of medicine, nursing, pharmacy, and social work (Keuroghlian, Levander).

NOTE: This list is the rapporteurs' summary of points made by the individual speakers identified, and the statements have not been endorsed or verified by the National Academies of Sciences, Engineering, and Medicine. They are not intended to reflect a consensus among workshop participants.

4

Current Federal Priorities and Regulatory Flexibilities during the COVID-19 Pandemic

HIGHLIGHTS

- Only about 1 in 10 people who need treatment for opioid use disorder (OUD) receive treatment at an opioid treatment program (OTP). Barriers include an insufficient number of OTPs, their lack of integration with health care delivery systems, the fact that some do not offer all three approved medications for OUD or accept Medicaid, and the punitive approach to treatment taken by some (Gupta).
- Methadone has been shown to reduce opioid cravings, illicit opioid use, and risk of overdose, while also increasing retention; however, it is the least readily available of the three Food and Drug Administration–approved medications to treat opioid use disorder (Haffajee).
- In response to the COVID-19 pandemic and escalating overdose harms, the U.S. Department of Health and Human Services increased investments to address the opioid crisis (Haffajee).
- Different interpretations by states and OTP directors of regulations defined in Title 42 of the Code of Federal Regulations Part 8 have resulted in variations in how rules are implemented at OTPs, particularly regarding how frequently patients can receive methadone, as well what they must do to qualify for take-home doses (Olsen).

- In response to the COVID-19 pandemic, the Substance Abuse and Mental Health Services Administration, Drug Enforcement Administration, and Centers for Medicare & Medicaid Services have issued exceptions to regulations impacting OTPs, enabling a broader use of take-homes; the use of telehealth for check-ins, counseling, and peer support; and use of mobile medication units (Olsen, O'Malley).
- Although take-home regulations were eased in response to the pandemic, there was a lack of consensus around who should be eligible for longer take-homes. A minority of patients with OUD received extended take-homes doses of 14 or 28 days (Krawczyk).
- Stigma around the use of methadone limits the potential impact of regulatory changes and needs to be addressed both in the general population and among health care professionals (Olsen).
- Research indicates that relaxed take-home restrictions have had little effect on diversion, overdose deaths, or methadone-related poisonings, and have improved patients' autonomy, independence, and feelings of normalcy (Krawczyk).
- Federal regulations are implemented unevenly across states and OTPs, resulting in wide divergence across the country in the number of OTPs operating, the availability of take-homes doses and the definition of stability for take-homes doses, whether patients can be discharged for violating program rules, counseling requirements, and frequency of drug screening (McGaffey).

NOTE: This list is the rapporteurs' summary of points made by the individual speakers identified, and the statements have not been endorsed or verified by the National Academies of Sciences, Engineering, and Medicine. They are not intended to reflect a consensus among workshop participants.

The opioid overdose crisis worsened during the COVID-19 pandemic, especially among racially minoritized population groups, as noted by Magdalena Cerdá in Chapter 3. The presence in many communities of the powerful synthetic opioid fentanyl has driven much of this increase, said Rahul Gupta. Compounding this is the fact that people are not able to access the addiction treatment they need, he added. "In 2020, only 1 out of 10 people who needed treatment for illicit drug use received it at a specialized facility," said Gupta (SAMHSA, 2021). There simply are not enough opioid treatment programs (OPTs) available, he said, and many of the OTPs that exist are facing challenges in providing care. These challenges arise first from the fact that OTPs historically have been siloed from health care delivery systems. In addition, some do not offer all three forms of medication for opioid use disorder (OUD), not all of them accept Medicaid, and some take a punitive approach to treatment, said Gupta.

GOALS AND PRIORITIES OF THE CURRENT ADMINISTRATION

In March 2021, President Biden signed into law the American Rescue Plan Act,[1] which invested nearly $4 billion in expanding access to vital mental health and substance use disorder services, said Gupta. First-year policy priorities included reviewing methadone treatment policies and modernizing the way methadone is used.

The President's inaugural national drug strategy[2] also prioritizes expanding access to quality treatment and reducing racial inequities related to addiction, especially in health care and the criminal justice system. "We need to build a system of care that proactively seeks to diagnose and treat individuals, rather than waiting until they come into the criminal justice system or present with an overdose," said Gupta. He also advocated exploring what the federal government can do to help OTPs become more culturally and linguistically competent and more accessible to all, including by accepting insurance.

Gupta added that while evidence-based treatment can save lives, stigma often prevents people from getting the help they need. He compared attitudes about addiction today to attitudes about cancer in the past. With the formation of the American Cancer Society in 1913, he said, "Our country leaned into this. We made sure that we advocated for change, we improved treatments, and today cancer is a disease that receives more attention and funding than just about anything else." Not only are more treatments now available, but a diagnosis of cancer engenders compassion rather than blame. "Yet, that is not the case for the disease of addiction," he said.

---

[1] For more information about the American Rescue Plan Act of 2021, go to https://www.congress.gov/bill/117th-congress/house-bill/1319 (accessed May 6, 2022).

[2] The Biden Administration's National Drug Control Strategy was released soon after this workshop was held and is available at https://www.whitehouse.gov/wp-content/uploads/2022/04/National-Drug-Control-2022Strategy.pdf (accessed May 2, 2022).

The U.S. Department of Health and Human Services Response to the Opioid Crisis

Of the three approved medications to treat OUD, methadone is the least easily prescribed, despite the fact that decades of research show that it effectively reduces opioid cravings, illicit opioid use, and risk of opioid overdose, and increases rates of treatment retention, said Rebecca Haffajee, Acting Assistant Secretary for Planning and Evaluation and Principal Deputy Assistant Secretary for Planning and Evaluation at the U.S. Department of Health and Human Services (HHS) (see Figure 4-1). Given the escalating opioid crisis, experts across HHS came together in 2021 to leverage the best evidence available and devise a new overdose prevention strategy,[3] said Haffajee. This strategy identified four key target areas: (1) primary prevention, harm reduction, evidence-based treatment, and recovery support; (2) four crosscutting principles: equity, coordination, collaboration, and integration; (3) data and evidence; and (4) reducing stigma. Haffajee

MOUD	OTPs	DATA-Waivered Providers	Any Prescriber
Methadone	Yes	No	No
Buprenorphine	Yes	Yes	No
Naltrexone	Yes	Yes	Yes

FIGURE 4-1 Evidence-based medications to treat opioid use disorder. Despite evidence showing that methadone reduces opioid cravings, illicit opioid use, and risk of overdose, while also increasing retention, it is the least readily available of the three approved MOUDs.
NOTE: DATA = Drug Addiction Treatment Act; MOUD = medications for opioid use disorder; OTPs = opioid treatment programs.
SOURCE: Presented by Rebecca Haffajee, March 3, 2022.

---

[3] To learn more about the HHS Overdose Prevention Strategy, go to https://www.hhs.gov/overdose-prevention (accessed April 5, 2022).

noted that this strategy differs from the approach taken by the previous administration by shifting the focus to overdose rather than opioids alone and by taking a life span and continuum-of-care approach, with integration across sectors and types of care.

To close the gap between research and care, HHS is also substantially increasing investments to address overdose above and beyond the increases in funding seen in response to the COVID-19 pandemic, said Haffajee. For example, she cited the National Institute on Drug Abuse's (NIDA's) medication development program, which has funded research on the long-acting formulation of methadone that has received fast-track Food and Drug Administration (FDA) designation. "This formulation has the potential to increase treatment, uptake, adherence, and retention," said Haffajee. She added that NIDA's Clinical Trials Network[4] is also supporting development of innovations such as remote monitoring of methadone ingestion and incorporating pharmacists into collaborative care models.

As part of the National Institutes of Health (NIH) Helping to End Addiction Long-Term (HEAL) Initiative, NIH has also launched the HEALing Communities Study,[5] which is testing the integration of prevention, overdose treatment, and medication-based treatment at an array of settings (e.g., primary care, emergency department, community settings) in 67 urban and rural communities across 4 states, said Haffajee. To address concerns about providing treatment for OUD within the criminal justice system, the NIH HEAL Initiative is also testing different interventions to enhance quality care through the Justice Community Opioid Innovation Network (JCOIN).[6] Haffajee noted that as part of that project, a survey conducted in 21 states with the highest opioid overdose rates found that methadone was available in only 9 percent of the 583 prisons managed by prison systems surveyed (Scott et al., 2021). Even when it was available, it was often limited to subsets of patients such as pregnant women, she said. One of the problems they uncovered was that while establishing jail-based OTPs was onerous and costly, transporting patients to local OTPs was equally as onerous and cost prohibitive, said Haffajee.

Also under the umbrella of HHS, the Center for Medicare and Medicaid Innovation (CMMI) administers the Maternal Opioid Misuse (MOM) delivery model,[7] a patient-centered service delivery model that is supporting

---

[4] To learn more about NIDA's Clinical Trials Network, go to https://nida.nih.gov/about-nida/organization/cctn/clinical-trials-network-ctn (accessed May 6, 2022).

[5] To learn more about the HEALing Communities Study, go to https://heal.nih.gov/research/research-to-practice/healing-communities (accessed April 5, 2022).

[6] To learn more about the Justice Community Opioid Network (JCOIN), go to https://heal.nih.gov/research/research-to-practice/jcoin (accessed March 5, 2022).

[7] To learn more about the Maternal Opioid Misuse (MOM) model, go to https://innovation.cms.gov/innovation-models/maternal-opioid-misuse-model (accessed April 5, 2022).

3,300 to 5,000 pregnant and postpartum Medicaid beneficiaries and their infants in eight states (Esposito et al., 2021). Haffajee said the goal is to improve quality of care and reduce costs, as well as to reduce fragmentation of care and improve care coordination, including with OTPs and medications for opioid use disorder (MOUD) providers. She added that since the beginning of 2020, OTPs can receive bundled payments under Medicare Part B for services that include dispensing of medications, including methadone, for OUD. Haffajee noted that the Substance Use-Disorder Prevention that Promotes Opioid Recovery and Treatment (SUPPORT) for Patients and Communities Act[8] also requires coverage of all three FDA-approved medications for OUD, with implementation of this requirement to be rolled out between 2020 and 2025.

Data from the National Survey of Substance Abuse Treatment Services (N-SSATS) suggests that there have been some modest gains in the number of OTPs and the number of clients receiving methadone in OTPs over the past few years, said Haffajee. However, she said, "There is still a dearth of capacity and there are wait lists associated with many OTPs." Moreover, there are additional barriers to accessing methadone in certain settings, such as in justice settings and long-term care facilities, she said. Lack of integration with other medical care, such as prenatal care, further hinders the provision of methadone to certain populations, said Haffajee. Helena Hansen added that adolescents are often overlooked for methadone treatment as well.

SAMHSA Efforts to Improve OUD Treatment

Beyond the HHS overdose prevention strategy, the Substance Abuse and Mental Health Services Administration (SAMHSA), an agency of HHS, leads public health efforts to reduce the impact of substance use disorder and mental illness. Within SAMHSA, the Center for Substance Abuse Treatment (CSAT) oversees key federal regulations governing OTPs, said Yngvild Olsen, director for CSAT. Waivers to these regulations, defined in Title 42 of the Code of Federal Regulations (CFR) Part 8,[9] have occurred in response to the COVID pandemic, resulting in significant changes in the field over the past 2 years, said Olsen.

"Up until 2020, OTP regulations laid out a strict, and many have said too strict, process for OTP medical directors to approve take-home doses of methadone," said Olsen. The basis for approval depended not only on the length of time a person had been enrolled in the OTP, but also considered

---

[8] To learn more about the SUPPORT for Patients and Communities Act, go to https://www.congress.gov/bill/115th-congress/house-bill/6 (accessed May 6, 2022).

[9] To learn more about Title 42 of the Code of Federal Regulations Part 8, go to https://www.ecfr.gov/current/title-42/chapter-I/subchapter-A/part-8?toc=1 (accessed May 2, 2022).

whether the therapeutic benefits outweigh the risks of providing the patient doses that could be taken outside the clinic. Many states and OTPs interpreted this risk to include the presence of any non-methadone-controlled substance or medication, based on drug testing. As was described by Walter Ginter and Abby Coulter in Chapter 2, this often resulted in patients either not being given take-home doses or having them discontinued, triggering the requirement that they come into an OTP almost daily to get their dose. Many OTPs also interpreted the regulations related to other services as requiring all patients to participate in counseling or face discharge from the program. Olsen said there have also been concerns about the use of technology in providing methadone, particularly in light of the 42 CFR Part 8 requirement for a comprehensive in-person physical examination prior to starting treatment with methadone for an OUD.

Following the World Health Organization's declaration of a global COVID-19 pandemic on March 11, 2020, SAMHSA, the Drug Enforcement Administration (DEA), and other federal agencies issued a flurry of exceptions to regulations impacting OTPs, said Olsen. Most significant, she said, was the blanket exception[10] that allows OTP medical directors to provide up to 28 days of methadone take-homes to stable patients, and up to 14 days for unstable patients, if the OTP believes they can safely manage these doses. Olsen said that over the past 2 years, 43 states and the District of Columbia have taken advantage of the blanket methadone take-home exception, although some OTPs and states reportedly have backed away from the exception. Olsen noted that SAMHSA also provides block grants and state opioid response program grants to ensure coverage for individuals who are uninsured or whose health insurance does not include the coverage benefit of methadone-related treatment services. Meanwhile, SAMHSA recently released guidance to extend the take-home medication exception for 1 year past the COVID-19 public health emergency to allow time for the agency to pursue more permanent rulemaking.

Another significant change brought by the COVID pandemic was the authorization made permissible by the Centers for Medicare & Medicaid Services (CMS) flexibilities on telehealth, and SAMHSA regulatory exceptions to allow OTPs to provide patients with counseling, peer support, and check-ins via telehealth. "Emerging data and my own experience demonstrate that the ability to connect with patients through different telehealth platforms have generally been positive, from OTP, clinician, and patient perspectives, although not a complete replacement for all services," said Olsen.

Notably, she said, SAMHSA elected to exempt the requirement for an in-person physical exam only for patients getting buprenorphine, but not methadone, at an OTP.

---

[10] For more information about this exemption, go to https://www.samhsa.gov/medication-assisted-treatment/statutes-regulations-guidelines/methadone-guidance (accessed June 7, 2022).

Since the early days of the pandemic, SAMHSA has made other changes as well, said Olsen. After DEA issued guidance on establishing mobile medication units, SAMHSA issued its own guidance on funding for such units and defining which services can be provided. With the new mobile medication allowance and federal funding to support them, some states have begun to work with accreditation bodies to establish these units, said Olsen. The goal of mobile medication units, she said, is to try to get methadone to people wherever they are, whether that is in jail or prison, rural areas, or residential settings where pregnant people might be receiving services, or through other substance use disorder services.

Even with these regulatory changes, other challenges and opportunities remain, said Olsen. The first of these is the stigma around methadone. "Despite 50 years of clinical and research experience with this medication, I can't tell you how many times I've heard patients say they need to get off that stuff, as Walter [Ginter] mentioned, because they or their mother or their sister or significant other has told them it's just replacing one drug for another," said Olsen. She said she's also had physician colleagues tell her they will not consider patients for a liver transplant or replace someone's arthritic hip, or treat their severe bipolar disorder, unless methadone is permanently stopped. Patients have told her how badly they have been treated by primary care providers and asked to have the OTP be their primary care home. Behavioral health specialists working in addiction treatment have told her they do not believe in methadone, although they view buprenorphine as an opportunity to help people with recovery. She said she has also heard of OTP staff behaving as if they do not believe in the benefits of methadone treatment in helping people with OUD stay safe and reach their goals.

"So not only do we need to address stigma broadly across the board, but the health care profession at large needs significant training around methadone," she said.

Another challenge that needs to be addressed, said Olsen, is how to optimize quality of care for people with moderate to severe OUD, who often present with "a complex mix of multiple substance use disorders, physical and mental health conditions, the effects of trauma and discrimination, and other factors related to social determinants of health." In 2015, SAMHSA issued guidelines that describe a framework for what a high-quality specialty treatment system that includes methadone within the context of 42 CFR section 8 might look like (SAMHSA, 2015). She said the agency welcomes feedback on these guidelines as well as on how to promote the adoption of these strategies at federal, state, and clinic levels.

Drug Enforcement Administration's Efforts to Expand Access to OUD Treatment

DEA is committed to expanding access to medications for OUD, according to Kristi O'Malley, senior advisor of the Diversion Control Division within DEA at the time of the workshop and now assistant administrator of DEA. As mentioned earlier, they have temporarily lifted the requirement for in-person evaluation so that patients can receive buprenorphine prescriptions "issued for legitimate medical purposes" through telemedicine, she said. In coordination with SAMHSA, they have also waived certain parts of regulations for take-home doses of methadone to ensure that stable patients "can receive medication even if they are unable to leave their homes," said O'Malley, and they have promulgated regulations to implement a provision of the SUPPORT Act, which authorizes a pharmacy to deliver a controlled substance to an administering practitioner for the purposes of providing MOUD. She said "this step forward in patient care streamlines the process, because previously a patient needed to get the medication dispensed at the pharmacy, take it to the treatment provider, and then get it administered, and now that step has been removed." In July 2021, DEA also passed a regulation that allows the expansion of mobile narcotic treatment programs by "allowing DEA registrants who are authorized to dispense methadone for OUD to implement a mobile component to their registration, eliminating the separate registration requirement." She added that they have been working with SAMHSA and the Bureau of Prisons (BOP) to help provide people who are incarcerated with OUD with more access to methadone through a potential hub and spoke model making the narcotic treatment programs the hub and medication units with the prison the spoke.

O'Malley said that when DEA takes action against physicians illegally prescribing narcotics, patients can be left with nowhere to go for treatment. Thus, she said, DEA has partnered with HHS in the Opioid Rapid Response Program[11] to make sure patients are able to get the services they need. She added, "We've done the same with pharmacies, targeting them in a positive way to make sure they get information and know DEA supports them supplying [MOUD] to those who need it."

---

[11] To learn more about the Opioid Rapid Response Program, go to https://www.cdc.gov/opioids/opioid-rapid-response-program.html (accessed May 6, 2022).

REGULATORY CHANGE IN THE WAKE OF NECESSITY: LESSONS LEARNED FROM COVID-19

Decades of research, as well as the testimony of Walter Ginter, Brenda Davis, and Abby Coulter in Chapter 2, confirm that strict methadone regulations have caused tremendous burden, stigma, and burnout among people with OUD, said Noa Krawczyk, assistant professor at the Center for Opioid Epidemiology and Policy at the New York University Grossman School of Medicine. "It's like liquid handcuffs," according to a qualitative study by Frank and colleagues (Frank et al., 2021). Or as one patient in Frank's study said, "When I was on methadone, I was like a double slave. Like you're a slave to the heroin already, and you're on methadone, you're a slave to the methadone and to the clinic."[12]

The COVID-19 pandemic brought about not only revised regulations around take-homes and telemedicine, said Krawczyk, but also an opportunity for her and other researchers to examine how these regulations affected outcomes among people with OUD. Among some 30 studies conducted across the United States, researchers have collected data from OTPs across more than 25 states, she said.

Implementation of Revised Take-Home Regulations

The first question Krawczyk and her colleagues asked was how new take-home methadone regulations have been implemented in practice. Although a survey of OTPs across the country, conducted by the Office of the Inspector General of HHS, found that nearly 90 percent of OTPs endorsed increased take-homes to some extent with patients, at least two studies indicate that most patients were not affected by the regulatory change, said Krawczyk. For example, Krawczyk and colleagues showed that 70 percent of the OTPs surveyed in Pennsylvania indicated that none of their patients were eligible for 28-day take-homes (Krawczyk et al., 2022). A study in Connecticut showed that while there was an increase in the number of people eligible for 14- and 28-day take-homes, still only a minority of patients were impacted (Brothers et al., 2021).

Studies also showed that OTP providers had mixed opinions and perceptions about methadone take-homes, said Krawczyk. These varied from

---

[12] During the open discussion period, workshop attendees were provided an opportunity to provide comments via an online chat platform. In this regard, Susan Staats Combs, co-owner of the Shelby County Treatment Center and Chilton County Treatment Center in Alabama, cautioned against the use of terms like "liquid handcuffs," which are hurtful and can increase stigma. "Patients need it to survive, and it does not need to be paired with handcuffs. Methadone treatment, as do other medications, helps keep people alive! 'Liquid life' is what it should be," she said.

one provider who said that trusting patients to manage their methadone was beneficial to the patient–provider relationship to another who believed strict policies were warranted because of the risk of abuse and the "huge liability" for OTPs (Hunter et al., 2021; Suen et al., 2021).

Several challenges and facilitators related to implementing longer take-homes have also been identified, said Krawczyk. Challenges included a lack of consensus or guidance around defining stability for take-homes, concerns about exacerbating already existing disparities (e.g., some people not having access to safe storage due to lack of stable housing), and implicit biases and previous experiences with patients that could influence provider discretion around take-homes (Hatch-Maillette et al., 2021; Madden et al., 2021; Peavy et al., 2020). Telehealth-related challenges included questionable sustainability of reimbursement and how this might affect continuation of remote monitoring that began during the pandemic (Hunter et al., 2021; Joseph et al., 2021). Facilitators cited by OTPs included leveraging multidisciplinary treatment teams to make take-home decisions and using pillboxes and other strategies to reduce concerns around safety and diversion, said Krawczyk (Dunn et al., 2021; Kidorf et al., 2021; Krawczyk et al., 2022; Levander et al., 2021a).

Impact of Revised Take-Home Regulations on Overdose and Diversion

Researchers also explored how changes in take-home regulations affected the incidence of overdose and diversion, said Krawczyk. Opioid-related fatalities have increased dramatically over the past year, most driven by the synthetic opioid, fentanyl (CDC, 2022). However, methadone has historically and continues to represent a very small proportion of opioid-related fatalities (approximately 5 percent), said Krawczyk (see Figure 4-2). Moreover, she said, methadone-related poisonings, overdose deaths, and diversion also changed very little following COVID-19 regulatory changes.

Impact of Revised Take-Home Regulations on Patient Experience and Quality of Life

In several qualitative studies, patients were interviewed about the impact of revised regulations on their lives, said Krawczyk (Harris et al., 2021; Levander et al., 2021b; Suen et al., 2021). She noted several themes identified in these studies: Longer take-home doses provided patients with greater autonomy and normalcy; however, individualized care was key because some patients believed more frequent contact was beneficial in certain circumstances. Some patients also reported that take-home doses supported patient treatment goals by increasing flexibility and independence.

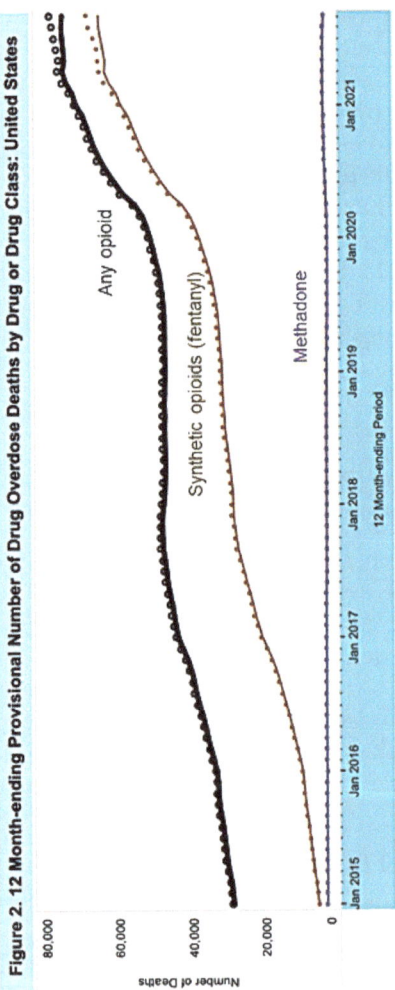

FIGURE 4-2 Twelve month-ending provisional number of drug overdose deaths by drug or drug class in the United States. Methadone (including for pain) continues to be involved in only 5 percent of opioid-related overdose deaths.
SOURCES: Presented by Noa Krawczyk, March 3, 2022; CDC, 2022.

Krawczyk added that there is little empirical evidence regarding the effects of regulatory changes on methadone retention. However, a study[13] conducted through the NIDA clinical trials network is under way to investigate this question, she said.

Policy and Practice Implications of COVID-19-Related Regulatory Changes

Given that recent research indicates that the new take-home regulations are safe and effective, Krawczyk asserted that the regulations should be sustained and expanded beyond the COVID-19 pandemic. "This type of individual flexibility should really be extended to all aspects of methadone treatment, including counseling and drug testing," she said. In addition, Krawczyk advocated for combining these reforms with other strategies, including expanding access to methadone via pharmacies, primary care, telehealth, and eliminating waiver requirements for buprenorphine.[14]

The majority of people in treatment for OUD, even in the United States today, still do not receive medication, said Krawczyk. "Increased access to medication in the criminal legal system is key for reaching populations that were historically neglected," she said. Moreover, she advocated ensuring that all licensed treatment facilities in the United States offer and encourage the use of evidence-based medications for OUD.

UNDERSTANDING THE DISCONNECT BETWEEN STATE AND FEDERAL REGULATIONS

As Krawczyk noted, federal regulations may fail to achieve their intentions because of how they are implemented across states and OTPs. Haffajee agreed that synergizing federal and state policies with regard to COVID-19 flexibilities is challenging, in part because SAMHSA provided the flexibilities but states had to opt in and provide the services. She added that while the federal government has multiple ways of declaring a public health emergency, all states have public health emergency powers as well. "It's a complicated rubric of different laws interplaying," said Haffajee.

---

[13] To learn more about the Optimal Policies to Improve Methadone Maintenance Adherence Long-Term (OPTIMMAL) study, go to https://nida.nih.gov/about-nida/organization/cctn/ctn/research-studies/optimal-policies-to-improve-methadone-maintenance-adherence-long-term-optimal (accessed May 6, 2022).

[14] During the open discussion period, workshop attendee Ruth Potee added that while she believes methadone should be prescribed by primary care doctors, just changing the regulation may not be sufficient, because less than 10 percent of primary care physicians have obtained the waivers necessary to prescribe buprenorphine, and far fewer actually prescribe it.

The Pew Charitable Trusts recently analyzed OPT regulations as of June 1, 2021, in all 50 states and the District of Columbia. Early findings from this review were presented by Frances McGaffey, an officer with Pew's substance use prevention and treatment initiative. To conduct this review, the research team coded state regulations and laws, compiled their results and sent them to state officials for verification. The work will be published as an interactive tool on the Pew website in Summer 2022. One state, Wyoming, provided no data as the state has no OTPs or related regulations, said McGaffey.

McGaffey highlighted some of the key findings:

- Twenty states restrict providers from opening new OTPs in some ways, either by requiring a certificate of need, placing a cap on the number of facilities that can open (one state, Indiana), or placing a moratorium on new OTPs (one state, West Virginia). McGaffey noted that restrictions on new OTPs contribute to long drive times to clinics, particularly in rural areas where the drive time is estimated to be six times longer than for people living in urban areas (Joudrey et al., 2019a).
- Although federal guidelines recommend avoiding administrative discharge of patients for violating program rules, such as for continued drug use, this practice is explicitly permitted in 27 states and prohibited in only 2 states, Massachusetts and South Carolina. McGaffey commented that research demonstrates it is safer to continue medication than to suddenly stop it (SAMHSA, 2020; White et al., 2005).
- While most states allow take-home medications during the first month of treatment, Pew found 10 states that prohibit this practice. Moreover, as McGaffey noted, "It's important to note that clinic policy matters here. Just because it's allowed by the state, that doesn't mean the provider allows it." Indeed, in a study conducted in collaboration with the Urban Survivors Union, Figgatt and colleagues reported wide variation in how clinics adapted to COVID-19–related flexibilities (Figgatt et al., 2021).
- Ten states also have take-home stability criteria that are more stringent than the eight requirements laid out in the federal rules, said McGaffey. For example, California requires that patients are employed, in school, a homemaker, retired, or medically disabled. "This limits the ability of people who might be earlier in their recovery, unstably housed, or just not in a position to be in school or employed from receiving take-home medications," said McGaffey.

- Federal guidelines require adequate substance use counseling to each patient as clinically necessary, but do not include a set counseling schedule. Nonetheless, McGaffey said 23 states impose counseling requirements and often tie them to the ability to receive take-home medications, despite research showing that strict counseling requirements can reduce retention in treatment and that medication without counseling can be effective (Hochheimer and Unick, 2022).
- Twenty-six states require more than the eight urine drug screens mandated under federal rules; 10 of these states require observation of sample collection, a practice that McGaffey notes can be degrading to patients. Moreover, she said urine drug screenings may not be necessary for patient safety, citing a Bronx OTP that suspended urine drug screenings because of COVID-19 and reported no fatal overdoses over the next 3 months (Joseph et al., 2021).

McGaffey concluded that in multiple areas, state rules do not align with federal requirements. One implication of this is that states could take steps to improve access to care even without waiting for federal action. For example, she said, Colorado recently changed regulations to remove non-evidence-based rules around urine drug screening, staffing ratios, and take-home medication.

McGaffey suggested that a more permanent solution might be legislation at the federal level, but acknowledged the challenge of issuing mandates versus providing flexibilities to different states. Moreover, she noted that changing federal rules around methadone will not be sufficient, said McGaffey. "Federal policy makers will have to work very closely with their partners in the states to make sure that changes are implemented on the ground and that patients actually receive methadone that meets their needs." She added that state policy makers are often unaware of the areas of misalignment with federal regulations. One of the goals of Pew's research, she said, is to raise awareness of the areas in which state regulations are not based on evidence.[15]

Individual workshop participants discussing current federal methadone regulations and regulatory flexibilities introduced in response to the COVID-19 pandemic offered potential ways forward to improve methadone access within the context of the existing regulatory landscape (see Box 4-1).

---

[15] For more information about the Pew Charitable Trusts' Substance Use Prevention and Treatment Initiative, go to https://www.pewtrusts.org/en/projects/substance-use-prevention-and-treatment-initiative (accessed June 10, 2022).

> **BOX 4-1**
> **Potential Changes to Improve Methadone Access Proposed by Individual Workshop Participants**
>
> - Building a system of care that proactively seeks to diagnose and treat individuals with opioid use disorder (OUD) (Gupta).
> - Developing policies to help opium treatment programs become more culturally and linguistically accessible to all patients (Gupta).
> - Adopting strategies that optimize the quality of care for people with moderate to severe OUD along with other physical and mental health conditions and social determinants of health (Olsen).
> - Developing guidance regarding the definition of stability in individuals with OUD and provide flexibility in determining take-home doses based on patient needs (Krawczyk).
> - Sustaining and expanding on COVID-19–related reforms by expanding access to methadone via pharmacies, primary care, telehealth, and in the criminal legal system, and eliminate waiver requirements for buprenorphine (Krawczyk).
> - Ensuring that all licensed treatment facilities offer and encourage the use of evidence-based medications for OUD (Krawczyk).
> - Improving implementation of federal guidelines by encouraging federal policy makers to work more closely with their state partners to ensure that regulatory changes are implemented (McGaffey).
>
> ---
>
> NOTE: This list is the rapporteurs' summary of points made by the individual speakers identified, and the statements have not been endorsed or verified by the National Academies of Sciences, Engineering, and Medicine. They are not intended to reflect a consensus among workshop participants.

5

Improving Access to Quality Treatment in Opioid Treatment Programs through Regulatory Innovation

---

HIGHLIGHTS

- In response to the COVID-19 pandemic, the Substance Abuse and Mental Health Services Administration (SAMHSA) modified take-home rules to allow states to request exceptions and provide 28 days of take-home doses for stable patients and 14 days for less stable patients, although the stability definitions were left open to interpretation (Dooling).
- SAMHSA has the authority to make take-home flexibilities permanent and could move quickly to do so by building a record showing the positive consequences of take-home flexibilities during the pandemic (Dooling).
- Layer upon layer of regulations and accreditation standards have resulted in opioid treatment programs (OTPs) that spend more time attending to regulations than caring for patients (Stoller).
- Accreditation requirements are components of many regulatory systems, but may create inequities in access to treatment and are not required by the Controlled Substances Act (Dooling, Parrino).
- There is a large and rapidly growing consensus regarding the need to increase access to methadone for opioid use disorder (OUD) both within and outside of OTPs (Schwartz).

- Current OTP regulations would allow using OTPs as a hub, with pharmacies, physician offices, mobile units, or other medication units serving as spokes (Schwartz).
- Pharmacy dispensing of OTP-physician prescribed methadone, along with other comprehensive care provided in an OTP (i.e., counseling, substance use testing, and monthly protocol assessments) improves patient satisfaction in stable patients who have been in treatment for at least 6 months and does not appear to result in a return to opioid use (Brooner, Wu).
- Community pharmacist-based dispensing of OTP-physician prescribed methadone could safely alleviate the shortage of treatment options for patients with OUD and improve patient access (Schwartz, Wu).
- Mobile medication units linked to brick-and-mortar OTP sites have extended the reach of medications for opioid use disorder, counseling, and other services in New Jersey and other states, including at correctional facilities (Mielke, Parrino).
- Hospitals can administer methadone to patients without involving an OTP if the indication is something other than OUD, but cannot initiate methadone treatment for OUD unless given specific authority to do so (Parrino).

NOTE: This list is the rapporteurs' summary of points made by the individual speakers identified, and the statements have not been endorsed or verified by the National Academies of Sciences, Engineering, and Medicine. They are not intended to reflect a consensus among workshop participants.

Federal regulations governing opioid use disorder (OUD) treatment, including the COVID-19 emergency allowances, have had both intended and unintended impacts, said Kenneth Stoller, associate professor in the department of psychiatry and behavioral sciences at the Johns Hopkins University School of Medicine. In addition, as discussed in Chapter 4, state laws may conflict with access and best treatment practice, he said.

The current opioid treatment program (OTP) system was established to provide a comprehensive approach to a complex disorder in a population that frequently has many social, medical, and mental health struggles in addition to misuse of opioids and other drugs, said Stoller. During the online open discussion period, Susan Staats Combs agreed, noting that many OTPs work earnestly to reduce stigma and help patients with an array of issues that led them to the clinic in the first place. "We help patients in every facet of their life," she added. Yet, regulatory constraints and a complex set of accreditation standards may stymie service delivery and limit access to certain populations, said Stoller. For example, these barriers can discourage the opening of smaller sized OTPs in areas of great need, such as rural areas. Regulations and accreditation standards have been added layer upon layer over time, creating a complicated multilayered system that results in OTPs spending more time attending to those regulations rather than caring for patients, said Stoller. By limiting access to "comprehensive, high quality, and safe treatment from well-trained professionals," he said, excessive controls could push methadone treatment toward unregulated and unaccredited office-based practices that would not provide the comprehensive treatment needed to help patients achieve recovery.

To improve access to quality and safe treatment for OUD, regulatory innovations are needed that are supported by evidence and best practices, said Stoller. Changes are needed that increase flexibility and make the opening of new programs and the operation of existing programs easier, while continuing to hold programs accountable for using the most proven and patient-centered practices and ensuring the safe use of methadone, he said. Among these innovations, pharmacy-based dispensing, mobile units, and expanding the reach of the OTP as a hub site are discussed in this chapter.

FEDERAL STATUTES AND REGULATIONS THAT GOVERN OPIOID TREATMENT PROGRAMS

The regulatory structures that surround policy issues presented by OUD and other pressing social problems start with the statutes produced by Congress, said Bridget Dooling, research professor with the George Washington University Regulatory Studies Center. These statutes provide federal agencies such as Department of Health and Human Services (HHS) with the authority to govern, which they do by producing regulations at the federal level, adding that Congress also creates and funds those agencies. Both statutes and regulations are law, said Dooling, but it is important to recognize that only Congress can change statutes. "On the flip side, it's a missed opportunity if we fail to recognize places where Congress has given an agency authority that it's not using," she said.

Potential to Extend Pandemic Flexibilities

With a grant from the Pew Charitable Trusts, Dooling and her colleague Laura Stanley have explored whether certain pandemic flexibilities such as those concerning take-home supplies of methadone could be legally extended after the pandemic ends. Dooling explained that the Substance Abuse and Mental Health Services Administration (SAMHSA) issues rules that govern how OTPs operate, and the rule is that patients must come to the OTP almost every day to get their doses. The opportunity to receive take-homes, she said, is the exception, not the rule. As Yngvild Olsen described in Chapter 4, at the beginning of the pandemic, SAMHSA issued a modification to the rule that allowed states to request exceptions allowing stable patients to receive 28 days of take-home doses and less stable patients to receive 14 days of take-home doses if the OTP believed the patient could handle these take-homes safely. The definition of "stable" and "less stable" were left open to interpretation, said Dooling.

"The pandemic shifted something fundamental," said Dooling, but understandably, people were concerned that SAMHSA would retract the flexibility when the pandemic ends. Dooling and Stanley set out to examine whether the law required that flexibility to end or whether it was a policy choice. "Our findings were stunning," she said. "We found that SAMHSA has a high degree of authority to make regulatory changes without going to Congress to change the law." Under the Controlled Substances Act, she said, the secretary of HHS has the authority to establish standards that spell out who qualifies for this kind of treatment. SAMHSA thus had the authority to make the take-home flexibilities permanent, said Dooling.

SAMHSA has stated that once the pandemic emergency ends, the take-home flexibility will stay in place for 1 year, said Dooling. "This will hopefully be enough time to get through the rulemaking process to make this flexibility stick," she said, adding that many studies have documented how the take-home flexibilities have worked in practice (as noted in Chapter 4 by Noa Krawczyk). "My advice is for SAMHSA to move as quickly as possible to build a record showing what we've learned from the take-home supplies available during this pandemic and to get a proposed rule as soon as possible," said Dooling.

She added, "The breadth of SAMHSA's authority also makes me wonder what else needs to be changed and how it should be changed to facilitate better patient care using harm reduction techniques." For example, the OTP model is part of the current regulations, but is not required by statute. She advocated for SAMHSA, the Drug Enforcement Administration (DEA), Congress, and state and local regulators to make it easier to pilot new ways of treatment. She also argued that bringing about regulatory change will require sustained attention with someone overseeing the activity, perhaps in the Office of National Drug Control Policy (ONDCP) or elsewhere in the White House. Noting that there are longstanding disagreements about the trade-offs between law enforcement and public health, this person should be a "deft policy maker who can guide the process, have hard conversations, and move the ball forward."

"We know so much more about addiction and opioids than we used to," she said. "Let's bring the reg[ulation]s up to speed so they aren't holding people back from the care that they need."

PHARMACY DISPENSING AS AN EXTENSION OF OTPs

When the regulations for methadone treatment were finalized in 1972, they made it illegal to prescribe methadone for OUD outside of OTPs, said Robert Brooner, a senior research scientist at the Friends Research Institute and emeritus professor at the Johns Hopkins School of Medicine. Yet, he said there is a large and rapidly growing consensus of the need to increase access to methadone for OUD both within and outside of OTPs. Robert Schwartz, a senior research scientist at Friends Research Institute, said an underused and often overlooked aspect of current OTP regulations is the possibility for an OTP to act as a hub, with pharmacies, physician offices, mobile units, or other "medication units" to serve as spokes.

Moreover, as Schwartz noted, dispensing and administering medication is explicitly what pharmacies do extremely well, adding that they are experienced in maintaining, storing, and accounting for doses of controlled substances. Given how quickly COVID vaccinations were brought to scale so quickly in pharmacies, Schwartz expressed support for using pharmacies for the delivery of methadone. Using the same dose administration and dispensing guidance as is used by OTPs, he maintained that medication and take-homes could be dispensed safely in pharmacies.

One important rationale for this approach is to mitigate a shortage of physicians specializing in treating addiction, said Li-Tzy Wu, professor of psychiatry and behavioral sciences at Duke University School of Medicine. She cited a 2012 study that demonstrated a substantial gap between those needing treatment for OUD and the treatment capacity available at that time (Jones et al., 2015) (see Figure 5-1). Wu added that licensed pharmacists are medication therapy management experts and are widely available even in rural areas.

Brooner has been working on a National Institute on Drug Abuse–(NIDA-)funded study to investigate pharmacy administration of methadone for patients being managed in an OTP. OTPs provide a natural laboratory in which to study how to collaborate with pharmacies as a bridge to making methadone more readily available even outside of an OTP, said Brooner.

Two small studies conducted in the late 1960s and early 1970s showed mixed results including reduced drug use, said Brooner (Bowden et al., 1976). More than 45 years elapsed before two studies of pharmacy dispensing of methadone were completed by Brooner and Wu (Wu et al., 2022).

Brooner's 3-month, non-randomized, single-arm pilot study was designed to evaluate the feasibility of having an OTP physician prescribe methadone and a community pharmacy dispense and administer it (Brooner et al., 2022). There were many delays in starting the project, said Brooner: about 15 months to obtain the necessary exceptions from DEA, followed by additional time to obtain the SAMHSA waiver, a support letter from

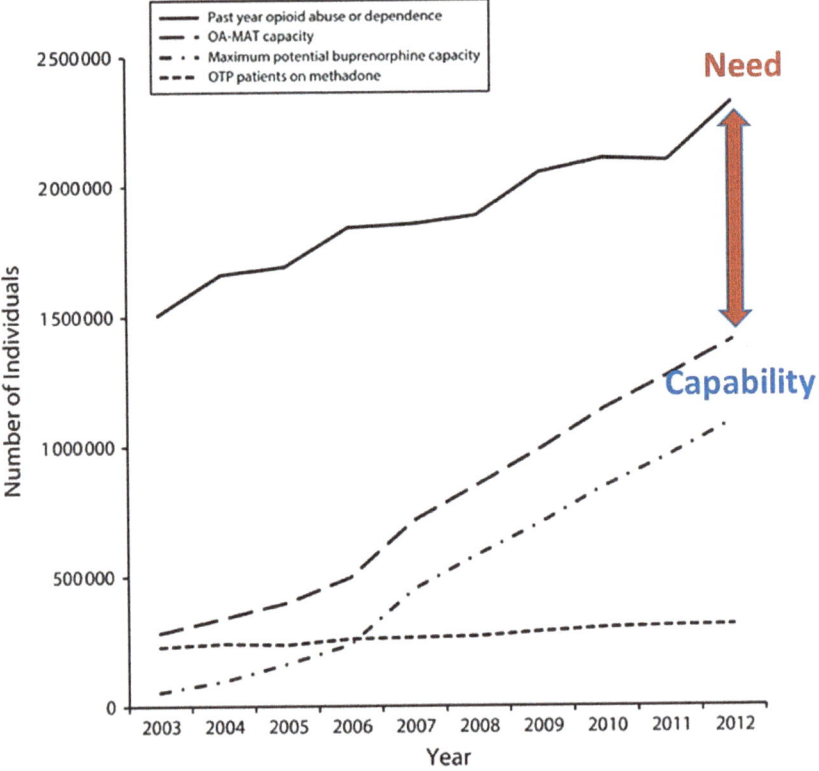

FIGURE 5-1 Lack of capacity to treat opioid use disorder. In 2012, the difference between the number of people with past-year opioid use disorder and combined methadone and buprenorphine treatment capacity was approximately 914,000 individuals.
NOTE: OA-MAT = opioid agonist medication-assisted treatment; OTP = opioid treatment program.
SOURCES: Presented by Li-Tzy Wu, March 4, 2022; adapted from Jones et al., 2015.

the state methadone authority in Maryland, and institutional review board (IRB) approval from Johns Hopkins University. By then the COVID-19 pandemic had shut down operations at many health care institutions, and subject recruitment was suspended for several months. Finally, in October 2020, recruitment began and was completed in less than 3 months. Patients were required to be stable, that is, on an unchanging dose of methadone between 20 and 90 milligrams for at least 6 months, able to demonstrate at least 80 percent attendance at counseling sessions, employed or in a community volunteer position, and between the ages of 18 and 66. Eleven patients were enrolled and 10 completed the trial, resulting in 91 percent retention. Participants self-reported zero days of opioid use and had zero opioid positive urine specimens; they also reported very high levels of satisfaction, according to Brooner.

Brooner emphasized that this study was conducted in highly stable patients who had long periods of abstinence. Additional studies are needed, he said, to determine if people with less stability and shorter durations of treatment would do as well. Federal and state approvals are needed to extend this work to other OTPs and conduct demonstration projects that enroll patient with shorter periods of stability and use telehealth for evaluations, counseling, and behavioral interventions, he said. Brooner also advocated extending this pharmacy-dispensing approach to office-based buprenorphine practices and projects where safety, implementation, and efficacy studies can be done. Brooner added that it will be important to work with Medicaid, Medicare, and commercial insurers to recognize prescribed methadone for OUD as an accepted benefit in pharmacy coverage plans.

Wu discussed another pilot study in which the prescribing OTP physician provides remote supervision of the patient's care, plus electronic prescribing, through a collaborative practice agreement. Wu's pilot study, described below, provides preliminary evidence of a potentially powerful way to expand access—a model that has already been used successfully in other countries, as is discussed later in Chapter 7.

Wu and colleagues have conducted two studies that demonstrate how a team-based care model pairing physicians with pharmacists may address access barriers to medications for opioid use disorder (MOUD). The first of these studies included three buprenorphine treatment clinics in North Carolina (Wu et al., 2021). For the 71 patients enrolled in the study, their buprenorphine care was transferred from their physician to a pharmacist for 6 months. During this time, physicians provided clinical guidance and/or coaching to pharmacists and continued to prescribe buprenorphine and determine dosage, while the pharmacists dispensed buprenorphine after checking the Prescription Drug Monitoring Program (PDMP),[1] conducted dose reconciliation and patient education, and monitored other health issues and safety events, said Wu. The study was very successful, she said, with very high adherence and retention, low numbers of positive drug tests, no safety events, and high patient and physician/pharmacist satisfaction ratings. Wu added that pharmacist compliance with checking the PDMP was also very high.

---

[1] The Prescription Drug Monitoring Program (PDMP) tracks controlled substance prescriptions to understand the behavior of the epidemic and to identify inappropriate prescribing trends. For more information, go to https://www.cdc.gov/drugoverdose/pdmp/index.html (accessed April 14, 2022).

Based on the success of this study, Wu and colleagues launched another pilot study to test a proof of concept about community pharmacy administration and dispensing of methadone, plus e-prescribing (Wu et al., 2022). She noted that while there are only approximately 1,800 SAMHSA-certified OTPs, there are approximately 67,753 community pharmacies in the United States (Qato et al., 2017). Leveraging the large network of community pharmacies could thus expand the number of methadone dispensing sites and address transportation and cost barriers that result in lower retention rates, reduced quality of life, and sometimes a patient's inability to keep a job, said Wu.

The pilot study had three components: a collaborative practice agreement between the pharmacists and OTP physicians, electronic prescribing of methadone from the OTP physician to the pharmacy, and a methadone visit checklist to document pharmacist-provided intervention and check fidelity. After receiving exemption approval from DEA, SAMHSA, and the North Carolina State Opioid Treatment Authority to allow prescribing of methadone, and from the Duke Health IRB to undertake the study, 20 patients were enrolled in the 3-month study. They continued to receive routine care at the OTP and returned to the OTP to continue methadone treatment after the study ended.

In terms of outcomes, treatment adherence was 100 percent, retention 80 percent (two patients withdrew because of work-related issues, one due to pregnancy, and one due to a non-study-related hospitalization), no illicit opioid use, 100 percent compliance with psychosocial counseling attendance, no safety issues, and 100 percent pharmacists checked with PDMP in all 207 pharmacy visits (Wu et al., 2022). Satisfaction among participants was also very high.

The next step, said Wu, will be randomized controlled studies, including in diverse populations and various geographical locations, comparing pharmacy-based and OTP approaches in terms of efficacy, effectiveness, and implementations. Changes may also be needed in policies regarding pharmacy and pharmacist training, accreditation, and payment for pharmacist-provided care involving methadone treatment, she added.

Pharmacy-based dispensing of methadone has the potential to also address inequities in the current system, added Ayana Jordan, an addiction psychiatrist and the Barbara Wilson Associate Professor of Psychiatry at New York University Grossman School of Medicine. Achieving this will not only focus on how to present the option [methadone] to minoritized communities including how to ensure methadone is consistently stocked and available, but also ensure that minoritized pharmacists and pharmacy assistants are involved in these discussions, she said.

From the perspective of an OTP owner, Susan Staats Combs noted during the open discussion period online that in Alabama, OTPs are required to have an in-house pharmacy, resulting in high costs and many hardships. While the in-house pharmacists are considered co-workers, she noted that the added issues of involving them in each patient's case, including granting them access to the patient's records and involving them in decision making, has been overwhelming and needs to be taken in consideration when considering pharmacy-based dispensing.

MOBILE MEDICATION UNITS—
A DEMONSTRATION PROJECT IN NEW JERSEY

In New Jersey, mobile medication units that dispense methadone are now available in six municipalities to extend the reach of OTPs, said Valerie Mielke, assistant commissioner of the Division of Mental Health and Addiction Services in New Jersey's Department of Human Services. The mobile vans (which are more like buses) all have DEA approval, are licensed by the state, and have separate SAMHSA certifications, even though they are linked and connected with brick-and-mortar OTP sites, she said. They were funded as part of the New Jersey Medication Assisted Treatment Initiative (MATI) through a $10 million appropriation to the Division of Addiction Services to make inpatient and outpatient treatment available for individuals with substance use disorder, said Mielke.

"It's an innovative strategy that enables us to deliver treatment services directly to the neighborhoods where they are most needed," she said. In addition, it allows treatment to be provided within the existing continuum of care and within the public health paradigm. Services are provided in a client-centered, recovery-oriented manner that values and respects individual choices and embraces the harm reduction philosophy,[2] added Mielke.

To receive services at the mobile vans, individuals must meet MATI eligibility requirements, including low income and a history of injectable drug use, opioid dependence within the past year, or a positive test for opioids, said Mielke. They also cannot be enrolled concurrently in another opioid medication treatment program or be under the care of a prescriber of suboxone, she added. Medicare, Medicaid, and some private insurance plans can be billed for services.

The MATI vans are able to provide outpatient services as well as walk-in care, said Mielke, noting that many individuals are referred by New Jersey's sterile syringe access program. People in residential treatment may also be referred to the vans. Some individuals receiving treatment through this program are also able to live in permanent supportive housing developed as part of the initiative.

---

[2] Harm reduction is a key pillar of the HHS Overdose Prevention Strategy. To learn more, go to https://www.samhsa.gov/find-help/harm-reduction (accessed April 9, 2022).

One of the mobile medication vans has been repurposed to dispatch and make medication and counseling services available to people who are incarcerated at the Atlantic County Correctional Facility, said Mielke. She said that Project Kickstart, now about 6 years old, has served approximately 1,600 individuals. About 1,400 of these individuals have been released from the correctional facility on MOUD and 82 percent of those individuals continued treatment at a brick-and-mortar clinic site after release, she said.

New Jersey's experience with mobile vans suggests that other states can consider initiating low-threshold, low-demand access programs such as in areas where individuals who are homeless gather or where individuals have difficulty accessing treatment, or in rural settings, said Mielke. These vans can also be a part of an emergency management strategy, she said. For example, during Hurricane Sandy in 2012, mobile vans were dispatched to areas where people were having trouble getting to OTPs.

Mark Parrino added that other states such as New York and Rhode Island are moving in the direction of developing van services. New mobile van guidance from DEA went into effect in July 2021. The next month SAMHSA sent a letter[3] to OTPs and state opioid treatment authorities indicating that funding was available for vans if OTPs were interested, he said. Because the vans may cost as much as $250,000 each with special adjustments and additions, this funding stream is critical, said Parrino.

Mielke's advice to states considering mobile medication programs included choosing a vehicle other than a bus because they found that if the bus broke down, services had to be halted. Instead, she suggested retrofitting a box truck with a separate cab, so that if something happens to the cab, another cab could be rented and services could continue. She also advised starting a public awareness campaign before introducing the mobile vans. Some communities did not want mobile vans in their neighborhoods and had misperceptions about the individuals served there. She added that funding is available for these vans because a recent guidance allows SAMHSA block grant funds to be used to purchase vehicles.

OTPs AS HUB SITES IN SYSTEMIC EXPANSION

According to Parrino, SAMHSA issued guidance in September 2021 outlining the kinds of services that could be provided through two different entities: (1) mobile vans functioning under the aegis of OTPs, and (2) non-mobile units, which are fixed site units. He noted that fixed site units need to be approved by state authorities, SAMHSA, and DEA, but regulations governing mobile vans associated with the OTPs, through the DEA

---

[3] To view the letter, go to https://www.samhsa.gov/sites/default/files/2021-letter-state-authorities-mobile.pdf (accessed May 9, 2022).

regulatory apparatus discussed by Kristi O'Malley in Chapter 3, do not need additional DEA approval—it is built into the process.

Parrino suggested that in addition to using a mobile van to extend the reach of an OTP, the OTP could also serve as a hub site with multiple vans acting as the spokes. He added that one of these spokes could provide access to treatment in correctional facilities if the facility wishes to engage in that opportunity, similar to the Project Kickstart program in New Jersey that Mielke mentioned.

To enable any of these innovations, SAMHSA and the state opioid treatment authorities will need to work collaboratively, said Parrino, because some of the challenges lie within the states. For example, state or county zoning ordinances may prohibit an OTP in certain areas. In addition, he advocated for states to adopt Medicaid reimbursement mechanisms that provide access to reimbursement for the full services offered through the OTP, similar to those adopted by Medicare. "This is not just a simple policy statement, but must be coordinated with the states and even within counties," he said. Moreover, he noted that the federal government needs to address OTPs' concerns that even if they wish to expand access, they may be unable to find trained personnel.

OTHER STRATEGIES TO EXPANDING ACCESS THROUGH OTPs DISCUSSED BY INDIVIDUAL WORKSHOP PARTICIPANTS

In addition to the approaches described earlier in the chapter, several individual workshop participants in this session considered other strategies that could help expand access to methadone at OTPs, as well as several potential regulatory changes aimed at reducing some of the barriers to methadone access that people with OUD may encounter (see Box 5-1).

Incentivizing pro-recovery behaviors. Stoller noted that contingency management, such as paying people for pro-recovery behaviors like attendance to treatment, has often been effective, but its implementation has been limited by provider fears that it could be considered in conflict with federal laws governing inducements for treatment. New Jersey has been looking into implementing such a strategy, said Mielke. Brooner added that because counseling interventions may take some time to become optimally effective, incentivizing the ongoing attendance of patients may help retain patients during this gap between delivery of service and patient recognition of its effectiveness.

Eliminating or changing accreditation requirements. Stoller suggested that accreditation bodies also play an important role in limiting access to treatment. Accreditation is used in many regulatory systems to transfer oversight responsibility from a federal agency, in this case SAMHSA, to a third party, said Dooling. However, she noted that there is no requirement in the Controlled Substances Act to use an accreditation model. She suggested that accreditation should be looked at in the context of the entire landscape of regulations in terms of how it works to serve patients. Dooling used the metaphor of pebbles in a stream to explain how individual requirements that may seem beneficial on their own can accumulate over time until they become onerous, in the same way that pebbles thrown into a stream can build up to block the stream's flow.

Parrino added that from the American Association for the Treatment of Opioid Dependence's (AATOD's) point of view, the requirement that OTPs meet onerous accreditation standards creates inequities because those standards do not apply to other office-based practices. "It goes to the issue of having [a] bifurcated system of care," he said.

Allowing hospitals and other institutions to initiate methadone treatment. Other systemic adjustments are needed to expand access, said Parrino. For example, Stoller mentioned that hospitals can freely administer methadone or other opioids to patients without involving an OTP as long as it is for no more than 3 days, or if the primary diagnosis for the hospitalization is something other than OUD. But hospitals, skilled nursing facilities, rehabilitation centers, and other entities cannot initiate MOUD unless they have specific authority to do so, said Parrino. Changing this would require DEA to work in conjunction with SAMHSA to modify the regulations on how they provide oversight, he said.

Easing restrictions for patients under 18 to obtain methadone. Stoller advocated eliminating the requirement that patients under 18 have two failed detox attempts. However, Brooner noted that in practice many programs have already moved away from these specific requirements and shifted closer to documenting only that the patient has a current OUD to be eligible for treatment. "42 CFR in those specific areas should reflect what the field already knows, and that is incorporate this more rational, reasonable requirement that we're providing, ordering, or prescribing methadone for a person who has a clear and present opioid use disorder," said Brooner.

Expanding exceptions to the 1-year history of opioid addiction requirement for patient admission. Stoller also advocated for expanding exceptions to the requirement that a person must be currently addicted to an opioid and has been so for at least 1 year before admission. He noted that there are only a few exceptions[4] to this requirement. Parrino added that this is

---

[4] Exceptions include "patients released from penal institutions with a documented history of opioid use disorder (within 6 months after release), for pregnant patients (program physician must certify pregnancy), and for previously treated patients (up to 2 years after discharge)." For more information regarding the federal guidelines for OTPs, go to https://store.samhsa.gov/product/Federal-Guidelines-for-Opioid-Treatment-Programs/PEP15-FEDGUIDEOTP (accessed May 9, 2022).

part of the policy recommendations AATOD released in September 2021,[5] which suggest that clinical judgment should be used to determine stability in treatment, but that the time requirement should be eliminated.

Expanding the use of telehealth and reducing the frequency of urine drug screens. AATOD has also recommended the use of telehealth induction of methadone through OTPs. Mielke agreed, noting that the expanded use of telehealth during the pandemic as well as relaxation of the frequency of urine drug screens resulted in more patients accessing OTP services and staying in treatment. "I think the most important thing is getting individuals into treatment and helping support their recovery," she said.

BOX 5-1
Potential Changes to OTP Regulations Proposed by Individual Workshop Participants

- Expanding exceptions to the requirement that a person must be currently addicted to an opioid and has been so for at least 1 year in order to receive methadone (Stoller).
- Eliminating the requirement that patients under 18 must have had two failed detox attempts before receiving methadone (Stoller).
- Extending take-home flexibilities instituted by the Substance Abuse and Mental Health Services Administration as soon as possible (Dooling, Stoller).
- Obtaining federal and state approvals to conduct demonstration projects on pharmacy dispensing and telehealth evaluations, counseling, and behavioral interventions to more patients (Brooner).
- Working with the Centers for Medicare & Medicaid Services and commercial insurers to recognize methadone for opioid use disorder as an accepted benefit in pharmacy coverage plans (Brooner).
- Adopting Medicaid reimbursement mechanisms in all states to provide access to reimbursement for full services offered through an opioid treatment program (OTP) (Parrino).
- Allowing telehealth induction of methadone treatment through OTPs (Parrino).
- Relaxing the frequency of urine drug screens (Mielke).

NOTE: This list is the rapporteurs' summary of points made by the individual speakers identified, and the statements have not been endorsed or verified by the National Academies of Sciences, Engineering, and Medicine. They are not intended to reflect a consensus among workshop participants.

---

[5] To learn more about AATOD's policy recommendations, go to http://www.aatod.org/wp-content/uploads/2022/03/Regulatory-Reform-and-Policy-Initiatives-for-OTPs-in-a-Post-COVID-19-World-09302021.pdf (accessed May 9, 2022).

6

Improving Access to Quality Treatment in the Criminal Justice System and Other Institutional Settings

---

HIGHLIGHTS

- A majority of incarcerated people meet the criteria for drug dependence or addiction (Gardner).
- Incarcerated people with opioid use disorder (OUD) tend to have more severe disease and are at high risk of overdose and death after release (Rich).
- According to data collected by the Jail and Prison Opioid Project, only about 10 percent of all correctional facilities offer any type of medication for opioid use disorder (MOUD), and of those about 40 percent offer methadone (Rich).
- Stigma is the primary reason that MOUD is underused in the criminal justice system, which is particularly averse to methadone in comparison to buprenorphine or naltrexone (Barrasse).
- Incarceration disrupts the supportive resources that could protect a person from overdose, so connection to community resources upon release is essential (Rich).
- The transition from incarceration to the community is a high-risk period associated with poor health outcomes (Wang).
- The Transitions Clinic Network employs people with a history of incarceration as community health workers to help patients navigate health care and social support systems upon release from incarceration (Wang).

- Minimizing the contact of people with the criminal justice system is the most impactful way to improve the health of people with OUD and could be accomplished through system-level changes (Wang).
- Limiting the use of MOUD in all parts of the criminal legal system is a violation of Title II of the Americans with Disabilities Act, although there are policy and practical barriers that can slow compliance (Barrasse, Dorchak, Rollins).
- Discriminating against people with OUD violates the Fair Housing Act and other federal statutes (Dorchak).

NOTE: This list is the rapporteurs' summary of points made by the individual speakers identified, and the statements have not been endorsed or verified by the National Academies of Sciences, Engineering, and Medicine. They are not intended to reflect a consensus among workshop participants.

The correctional system is the default health care setting when treatment for drug addiction has failed, leading to other behaviors, said Tracie Gardner, senior vice president of policy advocacy at the Legal Action Center. Indeed, she said, a majority of incarcerated people—some 58 percent of state prisoners and 63 percent of sentenced jailed inmates—meet the criteria for drug dependence or addiction (Bronson et al., 2017). Yet, she noted that correctional settings represent challenging environments for the provision of care. Consequently, the risk of death from overdose for people coming out of correctional facilities is extraordinarily high, she said (Joudrey et al., 2019b). Gardner added that improving treatment for opioid use disorder within the criminal justice system has the potential to provide more broad information about the care of people within the correctional system.

CROSSCUTTING REGULATORY ISSUES THAT IMPACT CORRECTIONAL FACILITIES AND OTHER INSTITUTIONS

While most of the world has figured out that punishment does not work as a remedy for addiction, Josiah "Jody" Rich, professor of medicine and epidemiology at Brown University and a 28-year consultant to the Rhode Island Department of Corrections, pointed out that the criminal justice system remains stuck in the punishment mode. As an example, he said, the United States spends $182 billion per year on mass incarceration, but only $2.8 billion per year on treatment for opioid use disorder (OUD) (NIDA, 2021; Wagner and Rabuy, 2017).

More than 2 million people are behind bars each day in the United States, about two-thirds in prisons and one-third in jail, and more than 10 million people cycle in and out of correctional facilities each year, said Rich (Minton et al., 2021; Zeng, 2020). He added that nearly one in five of these people coming in and out of prisons and jails have OUD (Bronson et al., 2017). Because jail populations turn over much more frequently than prison populations, he suggested that jails present an opportunity to provide treatment for many more people with OUD.

Individuals with OUD tend to self-report more chronic conditions, higher levels of disabilities, severe mental illness, or co-occurring drug use, and have involvement in the criminal justice system compared with individuals with no opioid use (Winkelman et al., 2018). Indeed, said Rich, the definition of addiction is continued use despite adverse consequences. With OUD, people develop tolerance and withdrawal, which leads to a cycle of ever-increasing dosages and often, involvement in the criminal-legal system, said Rich. During incarceration, their use generally decreases because of the decreased availability of opioids, he said. When they are released to the community, they have lower tolerance and are set up for an overdose. Consequently, people coming out of correctional facilities are at much higher risk of fatal overdose in the first 2 weeks after release, said Rich (Binswanger et al., 2007; Bukten et al., 2017; Ranapurwala et al., 2015).

He added that incarceration disrupts supportive resources that could be protective against overdose. "So what we have is the highest risk population at the highest risk time," said Rich, making it especially important to start treatment at this critical time. He advocated screening people entering the correctional system for OUD and either initiating treatment or continuing them on the treatment they have been receiving. Most critical, he said, is ensuring that they have connection to treatment in the community after release. "If we start people with treatment on the inside and have no provisions for them to get connected with treatment on the outside, we have not really helped them," he said. Rich noted that while racial disparities in the criminal justice system itself also extend to treatment in the community, he suggested that if high-quality treatment could be expanded in correctional settings and linked to high-quality care in the community, some of those racial disparities might be offset.

Medication is the gold standard for OUD in the criminal justice system as in other settings, said Rich. Rikers Island in New York started a methadone program in 1987 and until recently was one of the only such programs in the country. In 2016, he helped start the first statewide comprehensive program in Rhode Island, which offers all three medications—methadone, buprenorphine, and naltrexone—as well as linkage to care in the community. Patients and clinicians work together to decide what medication is best, said Rich. Surprisingly, when asked, most people knew which treatment they preferred: About half chose methadone, another half chose buprenorphine, and almost no one preferred naltrexone, he said.

Rich and colleagues have also launched a website called the Jail and Prison Opioid Project (JPOP)[1] that collects, tracks, and shares data about medications for opioid use disorder (MOUD) programs in prisons and jails and serves as a repository for resources on implementing such programs. Data collected by JPOP indicate that about 10 percent (n = 634) of all correctional facilities offer any type of MOUD and about 40 percent of those offer methadone, at least to some patients, said Rich. Most of these programs collaborate with an outside opioid treatment program (OTP) to get their methadone, but 19 operate as an OTP themselves. To operate as their own OTP is an onerous process, said Rich, yet he suggested that many of them already have a full pharmacy that distributes controlled substances in a controlled environment.

Figure 6-1 shows the treatments provided by the different programs. Interestingly, in light of the Rhode Island program's data showing that few patients prefer naltrexone, more than 200 programs offer naltrexone only. Rich suggested that the reason for this is that "naltrexone is a blocker so it appeals to the custody and control mentality, and it's a monthly injection." He added that people are generally started on naltrexone "on their way out the door" and that there is little evidence for it being successful in the long run.

In terms of regulatory changes needed to expand MOUD in correctional facilities, Rich noted that because regulations were not designed with these facilities in mind, many of them do not make sense. For example, he said, take-home doses are not an option for incarcerated people and some of the security regulations pertain only to facilities in the community. He asserted that a goal of methadone regulation revisions should be to encourage and facilitate expansion of methadone in correctional facilities and the connections to community programs after release. This is probably best addressed by revising clinical practice guidelines, he said. Other mechanisms Rich supports are reducing the obstacles for prisons to become OTPs, expanding how OTPs function in correctional settings, expanding the use of mobile units at correctional facilities, and enabling these facilities to have their own pharmacies with Drug Enforcement Administration (DEA) certification to distribute controlled substances. To expand community resources available after release, he advocated expanding the ability of pharmacies and physicians to provide methadone to patients.

Rich suggested developing regulatory structures for correctional facilities that parallel those used in hospitals, where people can be started on

---

[1] To access the Jail & Prison Opioid Project website, go to https://prisonopioidproject.org (accessed April 11, 2022).

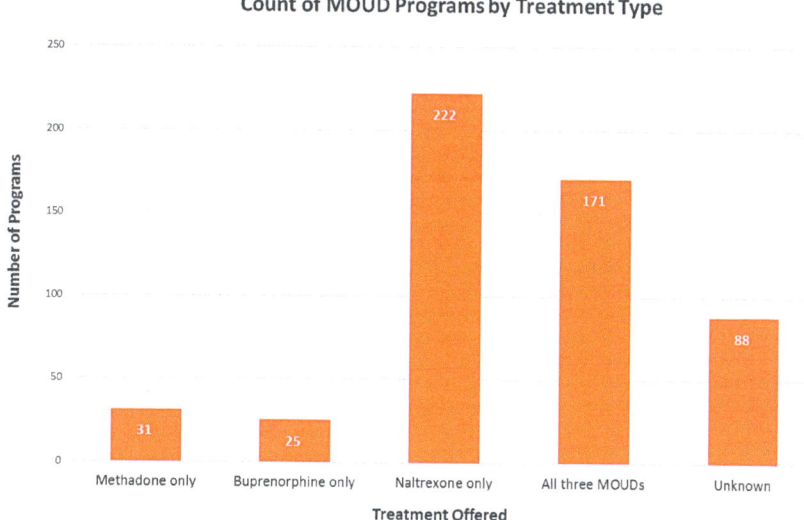

FIGURE 6-1 MOUD programs in correctional facilities by treatment type. Data collected through the Jail and Prison Opioid Project website indicates that most treatment programs in jails and prisons offer naltrexone only, although about 38 percent offer all three medications—methadone, buprenorphine, and naltrexone.
NOTE: MOUD = medications for opioid use disorder.
SOURCES: Presented by Josiah "Jody" Rich, March 3, 2022; Jail and Prison Opioid Project.

methadone, continue treatment, and link to community resources. He also recommended standardizing state regulations so they align with federal guidelines.

TRANSITIONING FROM INCARCERATION TO THE COMMUNITY

For people with OUD, the transition from incarceration to the community is a high-risk period associated with poor health outcomes, said Emily Wang, professor of medicine and public health at the Yale University School of Medicine and director of the SEICHE Center for Health and Justice. "A primary reason for this is that most return home without any access to safe housing, food, or gainful employment, and this is worsened by structural barriers that prevent people with criminal records from obtaining public assistance or applying for jobs," she said. They also have limited access to quality health care for a variety of reasons arising from the fact that correctional health care is largely siloed from community health care, said Wang. They may have to find their own doctor and reactivate their insurance, yet with criminal records, they face barriers to access, including stigma often exacerbated by racial discrimination, she said. In addition, parole and probation officers may prohibit them from being on MOUD. To help ensure that these individuals have access to primary care, Wang co-founded the Transitions Clinic Network,[2] a consortium of 50 community health centers nationwide.

The crux of the Transitions Clinic Program are community health workers, people with histories of incarceration, who help patients navigate the health care and social support systems after release from incarceration, said Wang. For patients with OUD, this may include providing naloxone, clean needles, referrals to safe injection facilities, evidence-based pharmacotherapy, and counseling, as well as addressing the social determinants that augment drug use: lack of food, housing, and income, she said.

As an example of how this approach can help recently incarcerated patients, Wang told the story of a 55-year-old man with a longstanding history of OUD as well as hepatitis C. He had been on methadone but was forced to detox from it when he was incarcerated and vowed never to do that again, said Wang. The Transitions Clinic treated his hepatitis C and the community health worker helped him navigate the bureaucracy to obtain food and housing. He continued to use drugs and when he was rearrested, the clinic made sure his hepatitis C treatment was uninterrupted, said Wang. Released again, he showed up at the clinic with cravings and asked to start MOUD. Since then, he received methadone and then buprenorphine at different points in time, is cured of hepatitis C, and works full time. Wang attributed this success by the medical home that allowed the patient to "engage in care how and when he wants, on his terms, in partnership with the health care provider and a community health worker."

Rich agreed that any kind of transfer in or out or between correctional facilities is usually the weak point in terms of health care provision and treatment of OUD. One reason, he said, is that people who are incarcerated do not know when they are getting out. "We tell people right up front, if you get out, go to the nearest OTP of this program (i.e., CODAC Behavioral Healthcare in Rhode Island) and they will dose you." Wang noted, however, that most people do not have the kind of robust OTP infrastructure that is available in Rhode Island. Rich added that there are many ways people can fall out of care, from not having a bus pass to losing their ID. "We need to try and facilitate retention in care after the transition," he said.

Wang added that while Medicaid restrictions, including the Inmate

---

[2] To learn more about the Transitions Clinic Network, go to https://transitionsclinic.org (accessed April 12, 2022).

Exclusion Policy,[3] contribute to the challenges for people transitioning out of corrections, this is not simply a Medicaid or methadone regulation issue. The point is to get people on methadone and keep them in care so they can thrive. "There are so many criminal justice policies that really constrain the patient's engagement and retention in care—collateral consequences such as bans on the ability to get housing, food, and employment," she said. In addition, as has been discussed by other workshop speakers, notably Magdalena Cerdá in Chapter 3, the most impactful way to improve the health of people with OUD would be to minimize their contact with the criminal justice system, said Wang. A host of system-level interventions could help achieve this, she said: minimizing drug testing; eliminating probation and parole revocation for drug use; lowering barriers for treatment with methadone, buprenorphine, and naltrexone; and providing strong social supports and resources for people to thrive in their communities when they return home after incarceration.

Bridging the Transition through Regulatory Action

Wang proposed several regulatory changes that might improve treatment of people following their release from incarceration and potentially help reduce the extremely high incidence of overdose and death among this population group.

- **Eliminate or modify the Medicaid inmate exclusion policy,** which prohibits the use of federal funds for medical care provided to an inmate of a public institution. The purpose of this policy was to prevent cost shifting to the federal government but is a major reason for the siloing of health care between corrections and community, said Wang. The Medicaid Reentry Act,[4] currently under consideration in Congress with significant bipartisan support, would allow Medicaid to pay for health care of eligible incarcerated people starting 30 days prior to their release, said Wang. This care could include methadone and other services, she said. The Act would also provide access to care coordination, enabling a smooth transition for patients, and create federal oversight for correctional health care that receives Medicaid funding, she said (Khatri and

---

[3] The Inmate Exclusion Policy excludes incarcerated individuals from receiving Medicaid. To learn more about health coverage for incarcerated people, go to https://www.healthcare.gov/incarcerated-people (accessed May 3, 2022).

[4] The Medicaid Reentry Act of 2021 is under consideration in the Senate as S 285 and in the House of Representatives as HR 955. To learn more, go to https://www.congress.gov/bill/117th-congress/senate-bill/285/all-info and https://www.congress.gov/bill/117th-congress/house-bill/955 (accessed May 3, 2022).

Winkelman, 2022). The Medicaid Reentry Act would also help bridge different payment systems such as Medicaid or other insurance, said Wang.

- **Create sustainable financing mechanisms for community health workers.** Wang said studies have shown that enabling Medicaid payments in correctional systems is a necessary first step, but not sufficient for engaging people with justice involvement into substance use or mental health treatment. Community health workers, especially those who have been incarcerated, are essential for building trust, eliminating stigma, and sustaining engagement of patients, said Wang. With stronger support, they could conduct "in-reach" into jails or prisons prior to release, meet patients, and coordinate release, she said. Data from the Transitions Clinic Network indicate that this in-reach approach substantially improves engagement. Multiple pathways within Medicaid are being explored as sources of sustainable funding for community health workers, said Wang.
- **Allow for methadone prescription and dispensation in Federally Qualified Health Centers (FQHCs) and pharmacies.** Joudrey and colleagues have analyzed drive times to the nearest OTP as it compares to drive times to FQHCs and pharmacies in five states with the highest overdose rates in the country (Joudrey et al., 2019a, 2020) (see Figure 6-2). In many counties in these five states, drive times to OTPs are greater than 60 minutes, but much less to FQHCs or pharmacies.

A STATE TRIAL COURT PERSPECTIVE

From the perspective of a judge who adjudicates cases of people with OUD charged with criminal offenses on the ground, the Honorable Michael Barrasse, president judge in the Lackawanna County, PA, Court of Common Pleas, the number one obstacle to MOUD in the criminal justice system is stigma. The criminal justice system is slow to change, he said. "It is adversarial and was never meant to be a change agent in dealing with behavioral health," Judge Barrasse said.

As an example of stigma and misinformation within the justice system, Judge Barrasse pointed to a lawsuit[5] recently filed in Pennsylvania, "The United States of America vs. the Unified Judicial System of Pennsylvania," in which the Justice Department claimed that Pennsylvania has "unlawfully discriminated against individuals with opioid use disorder in its court

---

[5] For more information regarding the lawsuit, go to https://www.justice.gov/crt/case/united-states-v-unified-judicial-system-pennsylvania (accessed May 9, 2022).

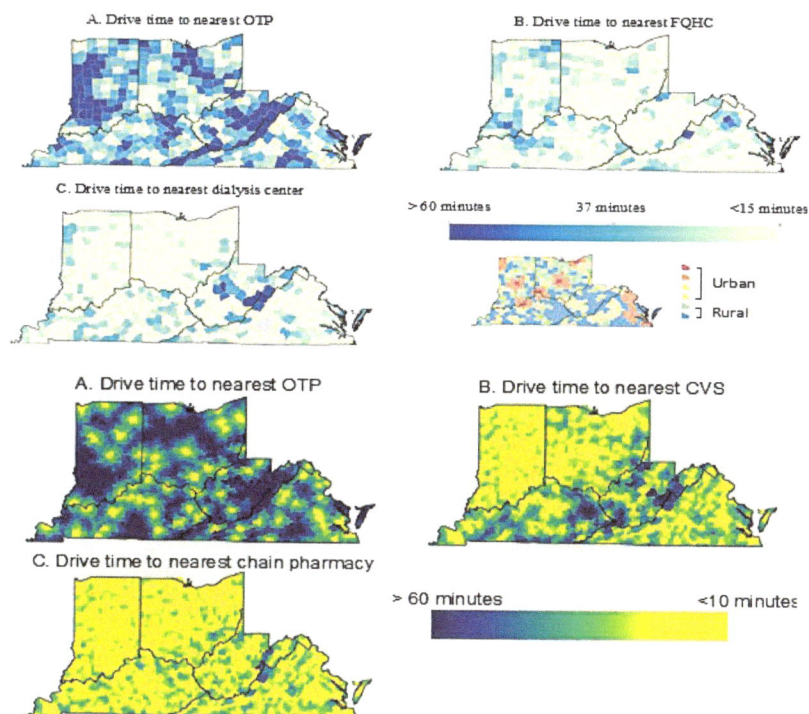

FIGURE 6-2 Drive times to opioid treatment programs as compared to Federally Qualified Health Centers (FQHCs) and pharmacies. The upper panel shows the drive time in minutes to the nearest OTP or to the nearest FQHC by county in Indiana, Kentucky, Ohio, Virginia, and West Virginia. The lower panel compares the drive time in minutes to the nearest OTP versus the nearest CVS pharmacy or chain pharmacy, also by county in the same five states.
SOURCES: Presented by Emily Wang, March 3, 2022; Joudrey et al., 2019a, 2020.

supervision program, in violation of Title II of the ADA, by prohibiting or otherwise limiting the use of medication prescribed to treat their disability." The complaint cited an administrative order issued by a judge for the Jefferson County Court of Common Pleas, requiring individuals under court supervision to be completely clean of any opioid-based treatment medication for 30 days or face revocation of their probation. The only exception was for pregnancy.

In issuing the order, the Jefferson County Court claimed, without scientific evidence, that "the vast majority, well in excess of 80 percent" of individuals who are prescribed opioid-based treatments, misuse those drugs regularly and that these treatments do not "appear to help the patients in any way to become productive members of society." The order further stated that "among the thousands of individuals who have been on probation while prescribed these drugs," fewer than 15 have successfully completed treatment.[6]

Judge Barrasse cited this case because, he said, it provides a clear picture of the problem. "If this is the mentality, and this is what the beliefs are for those people that are running the court systems, no matter how you change regulations, we are going to have a very steep hill to climb to make changes," he said.

Judge Barrasse added that the criminal justice system is particularly averse to methadone in comparison to buprenorphine and naltrexone. States have more restrictive policies for prescribing and distributing methadone, as well as inadequate pathways to obtain methadone upon release from incarceration, as has been discussed earlier. The vast majority of jails do not have methadone in their medication formularies and many local jails, which far outnumber federal prisons, have no MOUD under consideration in any form, said Judge Barrasse.

The criminal justice system depends on grants for funding, he said. He suggested two requirements for eligibility to receive federal grants:

- Individuals with OUD should be assessed for appropriate MOUD, including methadone, and a reason provided if they are denied. States, agencies, providers, and insurers who fail to follow this rule will be subject to prosecution by the Department of Justice Civil Rights Division for failure to comply with Title II of the Americans with Disabilities Act (ADA).
- Individuals with OUD deemed appropriate for methadone treatment should be provided with the same pathways to treatment as any other MOUD.

CIVIL RIGHTS LITIGATION TO ENABLE METHADONE TREATMENT IN INSTITUTIONS

As alluded to by Judge Barrasse, the ADA specifically requires that people with addictions receive access to treatment, including methadone, in jails, prisons, and other aspects of the criminal legal system such as courts,

---

[6] For an overview of the evidence base for medications for opioid use disorder, please see the National Academies' report titled "Medications for Opioid Use Disorder Saves Lives," available at https://nap.nationalacademies.org/catalog/25310/medications-for-opioid-use-disorder-save-lives (accessed June 12, 2022). The report concluded "FDA-approved medications to treat opioid use disorder are effective and save lives" and "long-term retention on medication for opioid use disorder is associated with improved outcomes."

parole, and probation, said Rachel Rollins, U.S. attorney for the District of Massachusetts. Yet, while disrupting treatment in the criminal legal system makes it far more likely that a person will commit further criminal offenses or overdose and die, Rollins said that 80 percent of jails and prisons in the United States do not allow methadone, and many court systems and judges have policies that prevent access to methadone. "Probation and parole boards sometimes go so far as to make not accessing methadone a condition of parole or probation," she said.

The ADA has been in place since 1990, yet Rollins said the first investigation into these unlawful practices was in 2018. Greg Dorchak, assistant U. S. Attorney in Massachusetts, said, "It took nearly 28 years before federal entities really started working in this, but now the tide has turned and they are enforcing it." He added that the ADA is not the only federal law that explicitly addresses discrimination against individuals with OUD. "So does the Fair Housing Act, section 504 of the Rehabilitation Act,[7] amongst other statutes," he said.

Dorchak said these statutes are designed not only to protect people with OUD, but also to address the barriers to providing treatment within the criminal justice system. He cited four ways that these laws protect the civil rights of people with OUD:

- Jails and prisons that do not maintain all three medications approved for OUD and provide them to individuals already receiving that treatment prior to entering their facility violate federal civil rights statutes, "just as they would have to be able to maintain somebody's blood pressure medication or insulin [for] diabetes," he said. He added that there are many ways they can provide these medications, for example, by contacting another entity that is an OTP.
- Parole and probation officers who order people off MOUD as a condition of their parole or probation also may be violating federal civil rights statutes when they are doing this as a blanket policy or practice.
- Skilled nursing facilities that refuse, as a blanket policy, admission to patients solely because they are on methadone or buprenorphine are violating civil rights statutes.
- Sober homes that reject people solely because they are receiving treatment with methadone or buprenorphine are violating federal civil rights statutes.

---

[7] To learn more about Section 504 of the Rehabilitation Act of 1973, go to https://www.congress.gov/bill/117th-congress/senate-bill/285/all-info (accessed May 3, 2022).

Dorchak acknowledged that while this may sound simple, there are many policy and practical barriers that can slow compliance. It might take a day or a couple of weeks to convince an entity that by law, they have to comply; then it may take as much as a year for the facility to navigate the complex system and actually provide methadone inhouse, he said. Dorchak noted that it can be particularly difficult for smaller, rural jails and prisons, where there may not be any methadone providers nearby or where only a few people who need methadone or buprenorphine go through that facility. For example, he said, there's no OTP on Martha's Vineyard in Massachusetts, so someone incarcerated in the county jail there would have to receive guest dosing from an offsite OTP as a more long-term solution is developed. Skilled nursing facilities have the same issues, he said.

"It's not so simple as flipping a switch," said Dorchak. "It requires complex decisions and can be a logistical nightmare" for entities to navigate these legal and logistical hurdles. Moreover, he said, most people do not know these practices and barriers are unlawful and that despite the complexity, they will have to comply.

Dorchak described another complication in the laws pertaining to incarcerated people with OUD: There is a carve-out in the ADA that denies protection for people illegally using drugs and an exception to the carve-out, which is that current illegal drug use does not apply to the provision of health care. For example, if a person entering a correctional setting takes buprenorphine but is also using cocaine, the cocaine in their system does not mean they lose their ADA protections for the buprenorphine because that is the provision of health care, which is still protected. "Legal acrobatics," said Gardner.

Rollins vowed that, as the chief federal law enforcement officer for the District of Massachusetts, she would make ADA enforcement a top priority and work with carceral facilities as well as nursing homes and hospitals to make all treatment options available and accessible. Moreover, she said, state departments of corrections and the federal Bureau of Prisons need to be educated about treatment of OUD and held accountable when they violate the law.

Potential strategies for improving treatment of OUD in and upon release from correctional settings proposed by individual workshop participants are summarized in Box 6-1.

BOX 6-1
Potential Strategies for Improving Treatment of OUD in and Upon Release From Correctional Settings Proposed by Individual Workshop Participants

- Screening individuals entering correctional settings for opioid use disorder (OUD) and start or continue treatment they have been receiving; and requiring compliance with this practice for correctional facilities to receive federal grants (Barasse, Rich).
- Revising clinical practice guidelines for treatment of OUD in corrections (Rich).
- Allowing pharmacies located in correctional facilities to dispense methadone and enable more correctional facilities to have their own pharmacies with Drug Enforcement Administration certification to distribute controlled substances (Rich).
- Reducing obstacles for prisons to become opioid treatment programs (OTPs), expanding how OTPs function in correctional settings, and expanding the use of mobile units at correctional facilities (Rich).
- Developing regulatory structures for correctional facilities that parallel those used in hospitals (Rich).
- Aligning state regulations with federal regulations on managing OUD for correctional facilities (Rich).
- Ensuring a connection to treatment in the community for individuals released from correctional settings (Rich).
- Expanding the ability of pharmacies and physicians to provide methadone to patients (in addition to OTPs) in the community after release (Rich).
- Eliminating or modifying the Medicaid inmate exclusion policy and pass the Medicaid Reentry Act (Wang).
- Creating sustainable financing mechanisms for community health workers (Wang).
- Eliminating probation and parole revocation for drug use (Wang).

NOTE: This list is the rapporteurs' summary of points made by the individual speakers identified, and the statements have not been endorsed or verified by the National Academies of Sciences, Engineering, and Medicine. They are not intended to reflect a consensus among workshop participants.

7

Expanding Access to Methadone through Regulatory Innovation: Envisioning Approaches Outside the Opioid Treatment Program System

---

HIGHLIGHTS

- Regulatory innovations outside opioid treatment programs (OTPs) are needed to improve patient access, alleviate provider capacity issues, and help address racial and social inequities (Jordan, Schwartz, Venner).
- Provision of methadone to stable patients at physicians' offices or pharmacies has been shown to produce high rates of treatment retention, a low percentage of positive drug tests, little diversion, and improved patient satisfaction (Schwartz).
- Managing methadone maintenance by physicians and pharmacists as an alternative option to OTP increases patient choice, reduces stigma, integrates care, and creates openings for new OTP admissions (Schwartz).
- Pharmacy-based dispensing of methadone has been widely practiced outside of the United States and may help address inequities in methadone (Nielsen, Sheridan).
- Access will require educating and supporting pharmacists to provide methadone treatment and ensure the availability of methadone in areas where inequities exist (Jordan, Nielsen, Sheridan).
- Training of pharmacists, pharmacy assistants, technicians, and other relevant staff is key to ensuring safe and culturally appropriate delivery of methadone to patients (Nielsen, Sheridan).

- Preliminary results showed expanded use of unsupervised dosing during the pandemic in Australia produced no evidence of increased mortality or diversion (Nielsen).
- Methadone treatment initiated at medically managed withdrawal programs (also known as detox), in inpatient hospitals, and in outpatient settings serving overdose survivors paired with direct admission to an OTP upon release, could reduce the high incidence of overdose and death among patients seeking care at these venues (Walley).
- In Black and Latino/a communities, community-based education, support, and coaching to address the social determinants of health as a path to successful recovery from addiction is essential (Jordan).
- To address the needs of American Indian and Alaska Native peoples, treatment programs should embrace a non-Western world view rooted in spirituality and traditional healing and should work in partnership with tribal communities (Venner).
- Compared to other racial groups, American Indian and Alaska Native peoples have less access to methadone as a result of regulatory and payment barriers as well as stigma (Venner).

NOTE: This list is the rapporteurs' summary of points made by the individual speakers identified, and the statements have not been endorsed or verified by the National Academies of Sciences, Engineering, and Medicine. They are not intended to reflect a consensus among workshop participants.

Throughout the workshop, participants explored opportunities to address current regulatory barriers to methadone treatment within opioid treatment programs (OTPs), as discussed in Chapter 5. However, several workshop participants also argued that this alone will not alleviate current access barriers to treatment, sufficiently increase provider capacity, and meet the demand for care. In this chapter, workshop participants explore regulatory changes outside the structure of OTPs—for example, office-based and pharmacy-based dispensing—that have the potential to further improve medications for opioid use disorder (MOUD), said Gavin Bart, director of the Division of Addiction Medicine at Hennepin Healthcare and professor of medicine at the University of Minnesota Medical School. Potential regulatory changes that could help facilitate these innovations noted by individual workshop participants are listed in Box 7-1 at the end of the chapter. In considering expansions beyond OTPs, Brenda Davis provided a note of caution, saying, "As we think beyond the historic integrated

OTP model where patients receive a variety of medical services, medication, case management, counseling, and other support services all in one place, it is critical that we not throw away the good with bad."

OFFICE-BASED METHADONE

Methadone treatment delivery in physician offices is not permitted in the United States without a Substance Abuse and Mental Health Services Administration (SAMHSA) exception, said Robert Schwartz. By contrast, he said, Australia, Canada, Great Britain, and other countries have permitted office-based methadone treatment and pharmacy collaboration for decades; office-based methadone treatment is available for stable patients as well as new and unstable patients, he said.

However, research on office-based methadone treatment has been limited, said Schwartz (McCarty et al., 2021). In the United States, "methadone medical maintenance" has been studied only in stable patients, he said. Among the advantages, patients experienced less stigma and had less interaction with drug-using patients, Schwartz added. He summarized published literature on office-based methadone treatment in stable patients from five case areas in the United States: Manhattan, Baltimore, the Bronx, Seattle, and a pilot study in rural Lancaster, PA. The minimum abstinence criteria in these studies ranged from 6 months to 5 years, although many patients had much longer periods of abstinence, said Schwartz. In Manhattan and Baltimore, methadone was provided by physicians, while pharmacies dispensed the methadone in the other three sites. The outcomes for these patients were excellent, with very high rates of treatment retention and a remarkably low percentage of positive drug tests, said Schwartz. To assess diversion, staff randomly called patients between visits and asked them to return unused methadone. All patients brought the correct amount of medication back to the clinic, said Schwartz.

Four randomized clinical trials comparing office-based medical maintenance to usual care at an OTP have also been reported in the United States (Drucker et al., 2007; Fiellin et al, 2001; King et al., 2006; Senay et al., 1993). In one of these studies, the physician's office was in the OTP. Schwartz said that in all of these studies, there was no significant difference between the two care models in terms of treatment retention or percentage of positive drug tests. One study also showed a non-significant difference in clinical instability, defined as two consecutive positive weekly drug tests or testing negative for methadone (Fiellin et al., 2001). In this study, patient satisfaction was significantly higher among participants in the office-based condition, although physicians noted that managing methadone administration was burdensome and better handled by pharmacists.

Another study was a three-group randomized trial comparing office-based medical maintenance, office-based medical maintenance in the physician's office in the OTP (rather than at the nursing station), and usual care in the OTP. Participants in the office-based condition received 28 take-home doses per month; those receiving usual care in the OTP got 5–6 doses per week (King et al., 2006). This study added treatment intensification criteria, where if a participant in the office-based condition had one positive drug test or one failed callback, they went back to the OTP for weekly counseling and drug testing and received only two take-homes per week. If they stopped having positive drug tests after 4 weeks, they were able to return to physician office–based visits and an increased number of take-homes. No significant differences were seen among groups in terms of meeting the criteria for intensified treatment, and most returned to their original treatment condition, said Schwartz. Participants in both office-based conditions reported significantly higher rates of new employment or social and family activities than those in the standard OTP group, he said.

Schwartz suggested several regulatory changes for new or unstable patients that could achieve the goals of increasing patient choice and increasing the number of people in treatment:

- Select and implement the best international approach for methadone medical maintenance using offices and pharmacies based on evidence of safety, efficacy, and impact on overdose deaths. The selected approach should include safe dose induction guidelines, direct methadone administration, take-home rules consistent with OTPs, and an evaluation protocol that compares outcomes to the standard OTP approach, said Schwartz.
- Leverage the Drug Addiction Treatment Act of 2000 (DATA 2000) buprenorphine waiver system[1] and community health infrastructure and link physician offices with OTPs or addiction treatment specialists to enable implementation of office-based methadone medical maintenance, he added.

For stable patients, Schwartz said the goals should be to increase patient choice, reduce stigma, integrate care, and create openings for new OTP admissions. To achieve this, he suggested:

- Expanding medical maintenance under current regulations using available evidence, and providing states and care providers with information about best practices, payment guidance, and how to obtain exemptions.

---

[1] To learn more about buprenorphine waivers available from SAMHSA as part of the Drug Addiction Treatment Act of 2000 (DATA 2000), go to https://www.samhsa.gov/medication-assisted-treatment/become-buprenorphine-waivered-practitioner (accessed April 14, 2022).

- Updating regulations to permit trained pharmacists with connections to office-based sites to administer and dispense methadone.
- Supplying methadone directly to dispensing sites to reduce bureaucratic issues and barriers.
- Aligning take-home rules for office-based sites with those used at OTPs.

INTERNATIONAL MODELS OF PHARMACY-BASED DISPENSING

The use of pharmacies for dispensing methadone (previously discussed in Chapter 5), while experimental in the United States, is widely used in other parts of the world, said Bart. However, the models used vary across countries, said Jane "Janie" Sheridan, associate director of the Centre for Addiction Research at the University of Auckland, New Zealand. For example, some jurisdictions limit pharmacy dispensing of methadone to only stable patients; some services require supervised dosing while others allow take-home doses; and costs to the patient may also vary, she said. Any type of pharmacy, ranging from independent small pharmacies to large chain pharmacies, may provide these services, although large pharmacies may have the capacity to treat larger numbers of patients as well as access to in-house training resources, which may not be available at independent pharmacies, said Sheridan. Whatever size pharmacy is providing services, she emphasized that they should have a private area for dispensing and good communication channels between pharmacists and prescribing physicians.

Small independent pharmacies may be the only pharmacies available in some regional and rural areas and should not be ruled out, said Suzanne Nielsen, deputy director of the Monash Addiction Research Centre in Melbourne, Australia. She added that if a large chain pharmacy decides to stop offering methadone because of its insufficient remuneration, this can have a major impact on access. Thus, she said, attention should be paid to reimbursement mechanisms and other types of financial support to encourage pharmacies to provide methadone programs.

Research and experience provide information about the benefits and issues for both patients and pharmacists of expanding availability of methadone beyond the clinic to community pharmacies. For example, patient access can be improved and allow more flexibility (Anstice et al., 2009), and may afford anonymity given that patients could be going to the pharmacy for any reason, not necessarily for methadone, said Sheridan. Pharmacists report improved professional satisfaction (Fonseca et al., 2018), including from developing supportive relationships with their patients, and there are opportunities for undertaking specialized training, she said. However, there are several considerations for both patients and pharmacists. Sheridan said patients report concerns about privacy (Neale, 1999; Neale et al., 2018), and stigma (Anstice et al., 2009; Matheson, 1998; Neale, 1999; Neale et al., 2018), and pharmacists have reported perceived concerns about safety, patient antisocial behavior (Fonseca et al., 2018; Matheson et al., 2002), and community resistance (Fonseca et al., 2018).

Training is key to ensuring the successful implementation of pharmacy-based methadone treatment, said Sheridan. This includes not only training pharmacists to recognize when a patient is intoxicated, for example, but also training around attitudes and stigma, and creating a safe environment where patients feel welcome. In the United Kingdom (UK), Sheridan had participated in "shared care training," where within a local area, primary care physicians engaged in training along with pharmacists and clinic staff around the delivery of methadone. Pharmacy assistants, technicians, frontline workers, office-based prescribers, and reception staff were also offered training and given the opportunity to talk about their concerns and misgivings about methadone. These types of training events, as well as improving professional networks, could, in the future, provide an opportunity to discuss issues around inequity and culturally appropriate responses to different groups of people, Sheridan added.

In Australia, around 80 percent of patients receive community pharmacy dosing and about half of pharmacies provide these services, said Nielsen. About two-thirds of patients receive care, including prescriptions, in primary care settings; only about one-third are prescribed opioid agonist treatments in specialist clinics. Medication is provided directly from the government at no cost to pharmacies but no payment is available to cover staffing costs to provide dosing, which typically means that pharmacies charge a dispensing fee to patients to cover those costs (Tran et al., 2021). A 24-hour help line provides clinical advisory services to both pharmacists and prescribers, and other clinical supports are also provided by the state to community pharmacies.

Methadone is listed as a "schedule eight" controlled drug in Australia, representing the highest level of control, but the same level as for morphine, oxycodone, and buprenorphine, said Nielsen. In terms of the regulation of pharmacy methadone supply, specific requirements around prescribing and administering methadone are usually outlined in state policies and clinical guidelines. While methadone prescribers are accredited in Australia, pharmacy accreditation varies by state, and individual pharmacists are not usually accredited, although they are recommended to complete training that covers jurisdictional policies and clinical aspects of care, said Nielsen. Lastly, the state health department must provide approval before a patient can start methadone (i.e., a patient-prescriber specific "permit" that limits a patient to one prescriber).

In addition to the regulatory protections, Nielsen noted that another aspect that supports patient and community safety within the community pharmacy program is the use of supervised dosing. She noted that early experiences in Scotland and the UK demonstrated significant reductions in deaths due to overdose involving prescribed methadone when unsupervised dosing was replaced with supervised dosing" (Strang et al., 2010).

During the COVID-19 pandemic, Nielsen said unsupervised dosing was more widely used and managed well. To mitigate risks of unsupervised dosing, patients are carefully assessed to determine the level of unsupervised dosing that is appropriate. A period of stabilization is usually required before unsupervised doses are allowed, and other checks and balances are in place, said Nielsen.[2] She added that some states dilute take-home doses to decrease the likelihood of injection (Lintzeris et al., 2002).

"To date we haven't seen evidence that it [increased unsupervised dosing during the COVID-19 pandemic] has led to increased mortality or diversion," Nielsen said (Coroners Court of Victoria, 2021), adding that unsupervised dosing requires targeting and flexibility. Sheridan agreed, adding, "It's possible to be more flexible without having disastrous consequences. The key is really careful assessment of each patient to see what is and isn't appropriate, and also making sure that each patient is receiving a therapeutic dose of methadone."

A naturalistic study in Australia found that dosing in community pharmacies rather than clinics improves retention; however, a study in Canada found the opposite effect (Burns et al., 2009; Gauthier et al., 2018), said Nielsen. Recognizing the limitations of observational studies, she acknowledged that patients were not randomized to pharmacy versus clinic dosing. She added that to increase treatment capacity in regional areas and use prescriber time more efficiently, Australia is taking steps to extend the use of pharmacists even more. This includes by enabling pharmacists to go beyond dosing to providing other aspects of clinical care. A model of collaborative care was co-designed with pharmacists, prescribers, and consumers, where pharmacists oversee treatment within a treatment plan, working within state and national guidelines with pharmacist providing reviews using validated assessment tools, she said (Nielsen et al., 2021).

INNOVATIVE MODELS OF INITIATION UNDER EXISTING REGULATIONS—INPATIENT AND OUTPATIENT SETTINGS

Even with the existing regulatory framework, there are opportunities not currently being leveraged to treat patients outside of OTPs before link-

---

[2] For more information on this guidance, go to https://www.health.vic.gov.au/drugs-and-poisons/pharmacotherapy-policy-in-victoria (accessed June 14, 2022).

ing them to OTPs, said Alexander Walley, professor of medicine at Boston University School of Medicine. Key to all of these "venue-based methadone initiations" is a trusting relationship between the initiation venue and the OTP, he said.

Direct Admission to an OTP from Detoxification Centers

At medically managed withdrawal programs, more commonly called detoxification centers or detoxes, many people seek treatment to reduce both their use of opioids and their overdose risk, said Walley. Yet paradoxically, detox is often followed by low treatment, high relapse, and high overdose death. For example, Walley and colleagues showed that between 2012 and 2014 in a cohort of 61,000 people in Massachusetts, MOUD treatment rose from 15 to 20 percent immediately after detox (Walley et al., 2020). In other words, most people do not receive treatment, he said. "This has implications because detox patients who do receive further treatment have better survival," as shown in Figure 7-1, he said, adding that in his opinion, "detox without further treatment really equals malpractice."

Instead of patients in detox being tapered from their initial methadone dose down to zero, they are titrated to control withdrawal symptoms and opioid cravings and then transferred to an OTP. Walley noted that these direct admissions will hinge on an existing, trusting relationship between

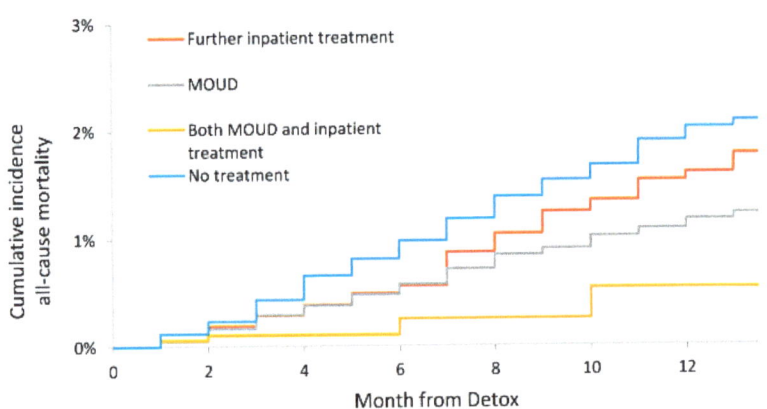

FIGURE 7-1 Survival in detox patients who receive further treatment. Mortality rates are reduced in detox patients who receive further treatment, with the greatest reduction among those who receive both medications for opioid use disorder and inpatient treatment.
NOTE: MOUD = medications for opioid use disorder.
SOURCES: Presented by Alexander Walley, March 4, 2022; Walley et al., 2020.

the detox program and an OTP. At least one OTP that must accept patients initiated and titrated at a venue outside the OTP. Many detox programs are certified as OTPs and provide methadone, and therefore can serve as methadone induction centers, said Walley. He advocated for this model and noted that all detox centers in Massachusetts with methadone on their formulary are certified as OTPs.

Hospital Initiation of Methadone followed by Linkage to an OTP

While only federally certified and accredited OTPs can dispense methadone for the treatment of opioid use disorder (OUD), an exception allows a physician to administer methadone to maintain or detoxify a person as an incidental adjunct to medical or surgical treatment of conditions other than addiction.[3] A study by Walley and colleagues showed that among patients who were initiated on medications for OUD or alcohol use disorder and then linked to outpatient addiction treatment, those linked to a methadone clinic achieved the highest rates of retention compared to buprenorphine and naltrexone through 6 months of follow-up (Trowbridge et al., 2017).

Delivery of Methadone in Outpatient Settings

A second exception to the requirement that only OTPs can dispense methadone for treatment of OUD is known as the "72-hour rule," said Walley. This exception allows a physician not specifically registered to conduct a narcotic treatment program to administer but not prescribe methadone or other narcotic drugs for the purpose of relieving acute withdrawal. Only 1 day's dose of medication at a time may be administered for no more than 3 days.[4,5] This approach was used successfully at a low-barrier substance use disorder bridge clinic in Boston in March 2021, said Walley (Laks et al., 2021). In the following 6 months, of 138 patients seen at the bridge clinic under the 72-hour rule, 129 were referred to OTPs, 4 were referred to inpatient, 1 was sent to the hospital, and 4 were already enrolled at an OTP, said Walley. Moreover, he said, among those referred to either of their two main OTP partners, 87 percent were linked to the OTP and 58 percent were retained at the OTP at 1 month (Taylor et al., 2022).

---

[3] Title 21 Code of Federal Regulations §1306.07 C.

[4] Title 21 Code of Federal Regulations §1306.07 C.

[5] A few weeks following the workshop, the Drug Enforcement Administration modified this rule to allow practitioners working in hospitals, clinics, and emergency rooms to request an exception allowing them to dispense a 3-day supply of medication. To learn more, go to https://www.dea.gov/press-releases/2022/03/23/deas-commitment-expanding-access-medication-assisted-treatment (accessed June 12, 2022).

Walley emphasized that all three of these venues see very high-risk patients. In another study, he and his colleagues have analyzed what they call the "critical encounter touch points" that lead to fatal overdoses. Opioid detoxification increased the risk of death 66-fold and non-fatal overdose increased the risk of death 111-fold compared to age-and-sex-matched individuals (Larochelle et al., 2019). "These are exactly the people that we need to make methadone accessible to because it is lifesaving and their risk is super high," he said.

Walley suggested five concrete actions that could facilitate better use of these venue-based methadone initiations:

- Issue and promote guidance for OTP direct admission approaches that already exist under current regulations.
- Incentivize partnerships between OTPs and detox centers, hospitals, outpatient clinics, and emergency departments.
- Transform detox centers into induction venues via regulation and funding incentives.
- Redesign OTP intakes to be welcoming rather than a "gauntlet" for patients through (1) true treatment on demand; (2) starting methadone for withdrawal within an hour; (3) liberalizing dose titration and take-home access; and (4) integrating methadone into the rest of health care.
- Fund research that evaluates innovative methadone initiation approaches.

POTENTIAL NEW TREATMENT MODALITIES AND SETTINGS THAT COULD BE OPENED UP WITH REGULATORY CHANGES

In addition to these innovative opportunities that could be realized under existing regulations or expanded with regulatory changes, workshop speakers were encouraged to "think outside of the box," said Bart. These novel types of settings provide opportunities to address racial and social inequities by making methadone more accessible, integrating community voices, and "lifting up the very people who have died unnecessarily during the drug overdose crisis," said Ayana Jordan. Potential changes that could enhance methadone access for racial and ethnic minorities noted by individual workshop participants are listed in Box 7-2 at the end of the chapter.

Culturally Responsive Community-Driven Substance Use Recovery for Black and Latinx Populations

Black and Latinx people with OUD are dying at disproportionate rates, and have less access to effective treatment, said Jordan. "This is a serious public health disparity that has not gotten the attention that White people have in dealing with their opioid use disorder," she added. Jordan and Chyrell Bellamy of Yale University are leading an NIH U01 funded study, the Imani Breakthrough Project, which is centered on the experiences of Black and Latinx people, with a focus on community-based participatory research and community trust. The name Imani, which means faith in Swahili, was chosen by Black and Latinx community members who said they rely on their faith to break through and access recovery in dealing with OUD and other substance use disorders, said Jordan. Imani Breakthrough aims to promote health and healing for people in the community by creating a sense of unity and collective responsibility, she said (Bellamy et al., 2021).

Part one of Imani Breakthrough involves a 3-month group education component, with classes and activities devoted to wellness enhancements delivered in Black and Latinx churches. "We talk about the social determinants of health, which SAMHSA calls eight dimensions of wellness—spiritual, emotional, physical, financial, environmental, social, intellectual, and occupational dimensions—that are needed for someone to be successful in recovery," said Jordan. In addition, a Citizens Enhancement Project[6] focuses on the roles, responsibilities, relationships, resources, and rights that are essential components of citizenship. Jordan said this project has been shown to decrease substance use without access to any medication.

The second part of Imani Breakthrough provides 3 months of wraparound support and coaching, provided by Black and Latinx facilitators and people who use drugs, to address vulnerabilities in the social determinants of health, said Jordan.

The U01[7] itself has three aims, said Jordan, who uses the term *medication for addiction treatment* (MAT): (1) to evaluate the impact of Imani plus a church-based, telehealth, MAT option; (2) assess whether there are changes in substance use over time for Imani plus church-based, telehealth-provided MAT compared to Imani plus traditional referral and linkage for MAT; and (3) evaluate potential mediators and moderators of improvements that affect primary substance use disorder outcomes; for example, how choice of MAT treatment location and social determinants of health affect whether people stay in recovery.

All Imani participants get the full 24 weeks of intervention, but 1 month into the treatment each participant decides if they are interested in medi-

---

[6] To learn more about the Citizens Enhancement Project, go to https://medicine.yale.edu/psychiatry/prch/research/comm_enhancement (accessed May 9, 2022).

[7] For more information about the grant, go to https://clinicaltrials.gov/ct2/show/NCT05260047 (accessed June 14, 2022).

cation; if so, they are randomized to MAT delivered via telehealth in the church or referral to MAT in the community.

"All of our services have been informed by and are delivered by people who live in the community, people with lived experience, and trusted collaborators," said Jordan. "We focus on harm reduction and choice, we emphasize mutual support, and we have intensive coaching to address the social determinants of health."

She added that Imani values community partnerships as a way of connecting with "diverse communities within communities." She noted that while being Black or Latinx has its own challenges, given the racism that permeates American society, "what extra stigmatization is added if you are non-gender conforming and Black or Latinx and have a substance use disorder and are engaging in methadone?" The different experiences of people with multiple stigmatized identities and the challenges faced by those who are undocumented or uninsured need to be better understood, said Jordan.

Jordan advocated for "#FreeMethadone" to increase access for Black and Latinx people and "reject the white supremacist organizing of methadone so it's only in OTPs." Her vision includes:

- Not requiring proof of insurance or other documentation to receive methadone.
- Allowing for telehealth prescribing of methadone in community settings (i.e., faith-based settings).
- Allowing for methadone to be given in primary care and community settings.
- Approving and extending the Opioid Treatment Access Act.
- Providing take-home dosing beyond 14 or 28 days when patients are stabilized.

Bridging Two Worlds: Methadone Treatment Consideration for American Indian/Alaska Native Communities

American Indian and Alaska Native peoples represent nearly 3 percent of the U.S. population and have one of the highest rates of opioid overdose mortality across all racial groups, said Kamilla Venner, a member of the Ahtna Athabascan tribe and professor of psychology at the University of New Mexico. She added that polysubstance use is present in many of these deaths. Most native peoples, about 78 percent, live outside of tribal areas, but about 22 percent live on reservations in tribal lands (U.S. Census Bureau, 2012).

Health inequities among American Indian and Alaska Native peoples are largely attributable to social determinants of health, said Venner. Lower median incomes, poverty rates nearly six times the national rate, and lower rates of achieving a high school diploma combine with discrimination, racial historical trauma, and systemic racism to negatively impact mental and physical health, which may contribute to the overuse of opioids, she said. Venner added that the Indian Health Service (IHS) is chronically underfunded. She also noted some positive health behaviors among this population, such as higher than average rates of alcohol abstention and vaccination. Venner attributed these strengths to the fact that the U.S. government allowed the tribes to align messaging on these issues to cultural values such as "save our elders who are the knowledge keepers," and "watch out for the community."

To address the needs of American Indian and Alaska Native peoples, Venner said that the Office of National Drug Control Policy (ONDCP) needs to understand and deeply integrate a non-Western world view rooted in spirituality and traditional healing and work in equal partnership with tribal communities. This means, she said, "deeply engaging them, taking the time to get to know them and learn from their great wisdom, and then investing long term with them." She added that the federal trust responsibility to Indian nations requires the United States to support tribal self-government and economic prosperity, protect Indian tribes, and respect their sovereignty.

Because of their sovereign nation status, federal and state regulations regarding methadone use do not apply to tribal nations, and different tribes have different approaches to treating OUD, said Venner. When dealing with a tribe that does not support the use of methadone, she approaches them with respect and a collaborative mindset to try to understand their position. If they are willing to engage in conversation, she may then have the opportunity to address misinformation about methadone treatment as well as the potential harmful outcomes when people are taken off methadone.

Venner suggested that there are aspects of evidence-based treatment that require cultural adaptation for American Indian and Alaska Native communities. For example, most evidence-based treatments are dyadic, involving only two people in the room, whereas a whole community may be involved in traditional healing. Evidence-based treatments are also stigmatized in this population, whereas traditional healing is admired; they tend to be secular rather than sacred; and they don't explicitly include native culture, whereas traditional healing preserves and values culture, said Venner.

"If we just offer evidence-based treatment without any cultural adaptation, it might be viewed as a broken bridge or something that is not inviting or maybe even treacherous," she said. "If we culturally tailor these evidence-based treatments, that bridge will look strong, inviting, and beautiful, and hopefully encourage more engagement and treatment."

Regulatory barriers discussed throughout this workshop may be compounded for American Indian and Alaska Native peoples, said Venner. For example, she noted that having daily in-person visits is challenging for people living in poverty; lack of privacy in receiving methadone can be stigmatizing and often is not humanistic.

National data also indicate that American Indian and Alaska Native peoples have less access to methadone, said Venner. For example, data from the National Survey on Substance Abuse Treatment Services showed that methadone was least likely to offered as a treatment for OUD if treatment was sought from an IHS clinic or if it was a tribally run clinic or a clinic with providers that speak the tribal language (SAMHSA, 2019). Facilities serving American Indian and Alaska Native peoples appeared to offer MOUD at typical rates, but were less likely to offer buprenorphine or methadone and more likely to offer naltrexone or vivitrol. Another survey showed that only 28 percent of facilities serving American Indian and Alaska Native peoples offered medication-assisted treatment for substance use disorder (Rieckmann et al., 2017). Payment barriers also limit access to methadone by American Indian and Alaska Native peoples, said Venner.

Venner suggested that to encourage engagement and overcome barriers of stigma within American Indian and Alaska Native communities, it may be helpful to frame methadone as a medicine and remember that they were some of the original pharmacists, using plants and herbs as medicine. She also advocated ensuring that providers, directors, and staff are themselves American Indian and Alaska Native or at the very least are knowledgeable and comfortable discussing culture; hiring American Indian and Alaska Native Elders as staff or cultural educators; and ensuring there is space for traditional services and cultural activities.

In developing such programs, Venner offered these suggestions:

- Consult and partner with American Indian and Alaska Native peoples.
- Learn from successful programs, such as the didgʷálič Wellness Center in Anacortes, WA, which offers all services under one roof, including administering medication in a private room and providing medical, behavioral, and dental health care.
- Advocate for more resources for American Indians and Alaska Natives.
- Make sure assessments are valid for American Indians and Alaska Natives and that treatments are delivered in a culturally centered, appropriate way.
- Increase the availability of treatments, decrease restrictions, and incentivize the delivery of methadone in humane and culturally appropriate ways.

BOX 7-1
Potential Regulatory Changes Beyond the OTP System to Expand Methadone Access Proposed by Individual Workshop Participants

- Replicating, and adapt when appropriate, successful international approaches for methadone medical maintenance in physician offices and pharmacies (Schwartz).
- Leveraging the buprenorphine waiver system to enable implementation of office-based methadone maintenance (Schwartz).
- Ensuring reimbursement policies adequately resource pharmacies to provide methadone maintenance therapy (Nielsen).
- Updating regulations to permit pharmacists with connections to office-based MOUD sites to administer and dispense methadone (Schwartz).
- Revising regulations for office-based sites that are in alignment with opioid treatment programs (OTPs) (Schwartz).
- Issuing and promoting guidance for OTP direct admission approaches that already exist under current regulations for detoxification centers, hospitals, and outpatient settings (Walley).
- Incentivizing partnerships with detoxification centers, hospitals, outpatient clinics, and emergency departments with OTPs (Walley).
- Transforming detoxification centers into induction venues via regulation and funding incentives (Walley).
- Prohibiting OTPs from requiring proof of insurance or other documentation for the delivery of methadone (Jordan).
- Allowing for telehealth prescribing of methadone and access in primary care settings (Jordan).

NOTE: This list is the rapporteurs' summary of points made by the individual speakers identified, and the statements have not been endorsed or verified by the National Academies of Sciences, Engineering, and Medicine. They are not intended to reflect a consensus among workshop participants.

BOX 7-2
Potential Changes to Enhance Methadone Access for Racial and Ethnic Minorities Proposed by Individual Workshop Participants

- Cultivating and valuing community partnerships to learn effective ways to study cultural adaptations pragmatically (Jordan).
- Addressing social determinants of health (e.g., unemployment, discrimination, transportation, childcare, housing, and neighborhood safety) that limit access to treatment (Venner).
- Incentivizing delivery of methadone in humane and culturally centered ways (Venner).

NOTE: This list is the rapporteurs' summary of points made by the individual speakers identified, and the statements have not been endorsed or verified by the National Academies of Sciences, Engineering, and Medicine. They are not intended to reflect a consensus among workshop participants.

8

Ensuring Equitable Access to Methadone by Removing Current Barriers and Providing Incentives

---

HIGHLIGHTS

- Regulations that require in-person dispensing at opioid treatment programs and limit who can receive methadone strongly impact access, but are not required by statute (C. Davis).
- Methadone flexibilities tied to the COVID-19 emergency declaration could be extended by tying them to the opioid emergency declaration instead (C. Davis).
- A carrots-and-sticks approach by the federal government could promote access to quality methadone treatment by relaxing requirements (the sticks) and improving payments and reimbursements (carrots) (Lawrence).
- The Center for Medicare and Medicaid Innovation has authority to test new payment models for methadone and roll them out nationwide if successful (Lawrence).

NOTE: This list is the rapporteurs' summary of points made by the individual speakers identified, and the statements have not been endorsed or verified by the National Academies of Sciences, Engineering, and Medicine. They are not intended to reflect a consensus among workshop participants.

In Chapter 5, Bridget Dooling described the statutes and regulations that determine how methadone is distributed and some of the barriers that prevent more equitable use of this life-saving treatment. Expanding on Dooling's remarks, Corey Davis, deputy director of the Southeastern Region of the Network for Public Health Law and director of the Harm Reduction Legal Project, stated, "Law is a barrier to methadone for opioid use disorder." But although the Controlled Substances Act prioritizes "ensuring that the wrong people aren't using the wrong drugs for the wrong reasons," flexibility remains regarding access to medications for opioid use disorder (OUD), he said. While both state and federal laws and regulations limit the use of methadone for OUD, he kept his comments to those at the federal level.

Matthew Lawrence, associate professor of law at Emory University School of Law, added that the federal government has tools that could be used to promote access to quality methadone treatment. He and Davis both suggested regulatory changes that could help achieve this goal. Their individual suggestions are summarized in Box 8-1 at the end of this chapter.

REGULATORY OPPORTUNITIES TO REMOVE CURRENT BARRIERS

The most important barriers to methadone access, according to Davis, are regulations that restrict dispensing of methadone to opioid treatment programs (OTPs) and the regulatory limits on who can obtain methadone maintenance treatment—only those who have had OUD for a full year and, for those under 18, two failures at detox. Regulations also require an initial in-person visit with a full physical work-up, limit initial doses, require periodic urinalysis, and set stringent criteria for take-home doses, said Davis. "And they apply regardless of the patient's needs and clinical indications and the provider's clinical impressions," he said. Indeed, during the online chat discussion at the workshop Zac Talbott, president of the National Alliance for Medication Assisted Recovery (NAMA Recovery), said members and stakeholders across the country are reporting the need for higher and higher doses for stabilization. One factor that may be contributing to the need for higher initial doses of methadone is the increased use of the powerful synthetic opioid fentanyl. Mark Parrino said most newly admitted patients are using fentanyl, "whether they know it or not."

The requirement that patients travel to OTPs to get methadone is particularly onerous, said Davis. As demonstrated by Kleinman, there are huge areas of the country where the nearest OTP is more than 2 hours away by car (Kleinman, 2020); see Figure 8-1. Therefore, even if other barriers were removed, the requirement to go to an OTP would make accessing methadone "basically impossible for people in large areas of the country," said Davis. He noted that the Drug Enforcement Administration (DEA)

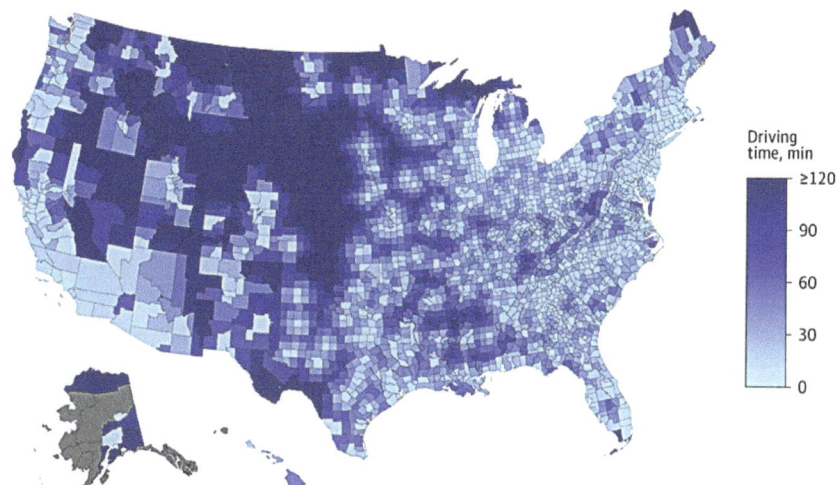

FIGURE 8-1 Driving times to opioid treatment programs (OTPs) in the United States. In areas colored dark blue, the nearest OTP is more than a 2-hour drive away for the average person in the community.
SOURCES: Presented by Corey Davis, March 4, 2022; Kleinman, 2020.

has made what he called "tweaks around the edges" allowing the delivery of methadone at satellite locations if certain criteria are met, but he maintained that most clinics lack the capacity to meet those criteria. Regulations do not permit OTPs to initiate treatment with methadone via telemedicine, even though this flexibility was extended to buprenorphine patients, who are more likely to be Whiter and are wealthier on average than methadone patients, said Davis.

As described earlier in the workshop, other flexibilities have also been introduced by DEA and the Substance Abuse and Mental Health Services Administration (SAMHSA) in response to the pandemic, such as mobile delivery of methadone and the availability of take-homes. While SAMHSA has proposed to extend the take-home flexibility after the COVID public health emergency ends, Davis noted that these extensions are currently slated to come with onerous requirements, such as total adherence to a treatment plan and negative toxicology tests for 60 days. Moreover, he said, none of these restrictions are required by law. "This is, in my mind, an example of the agency defaulting to the idea that our primary concern needs to be diversion and social control, not how to make sure that people who need this medication are getting it," he said.

Lawrence agreed, noting that DEA, with its focus on diversion, reports to the Attorney General and has veto power over the Department of Health and Human Services (HHS), which focuses on patient health. "So it's kind of a structural loading of the dice in favor of diversion as against other values," he said.

Ayana Jordan added, "The current situation is not working. People are dying at unprecedented rates" because of a shortsighted focus on diversion, which results in limited access. Available data show that when access to medication is increased, diversion goes down, she said.

Davis suggested that flexibilities could be extended by tying them to the opioid emergency declaration that has been in place since October 2017, similar to how they are currently tied to the COVID-19 emergency declaration. Both DEA and SAMHSA have the authority to grant exemptions to many methadone regulations and nearly unlimited enforcement discretion, he said, and they could relax enforcement immediately. Longer term, all of these onerous restrictions could be modified or removed through the regulatory process without congressional action, said Davis. Statutes require only that practitioners obtain a separate registration to deliver OUD treatments, he said.

The federal government could also take actions to improve the accessibility of methadone, said Davis. For example, Medicare funds nearly all medical residency positions in the United States and could require that to maintain funding, residents would have to be trained to deliver medications for opioid use disorder (MOUD). Similarly, funding of programs in the criminal legal system could also be tied to making sure people who want methadone are able to access it, he said.

REGULATORY INCENTIVES TO FACILITATE ACCESS TO QUALITY TREATMENT

Lawrence authored a commissioned paper (available in Appendix C) on federal administrative pathways the government could use to promote access to quality methadone treatment. In his workshop remarks, he focused primarily on regulations regarding permission and payments, likening them to sticks and carrots (see Figure 8-2): permissions being the sticks that regulatory authorities use to forbid doctors from prescribing or dispensing medications to patients, and carrots being the payments and reimbursements that attract providers into this space and enable them to continue and expand their operations. "We've spent a lot of time talking about the sticks, the limitations," he said. "But even if you take away the limitations, you're not going to see a lot of adoption if you don't have reimbursements."

Earlier in these proceedings, Dooling and Davis outlined the sticks side of this equation—the permissions required by the Controlled Substances Act and the broad standard-setting authority granted to the secretary of HHS, who delegates responsibility to SAMHSA, and the waiver authority granted to the attorney general, who delegates authority to DEA.

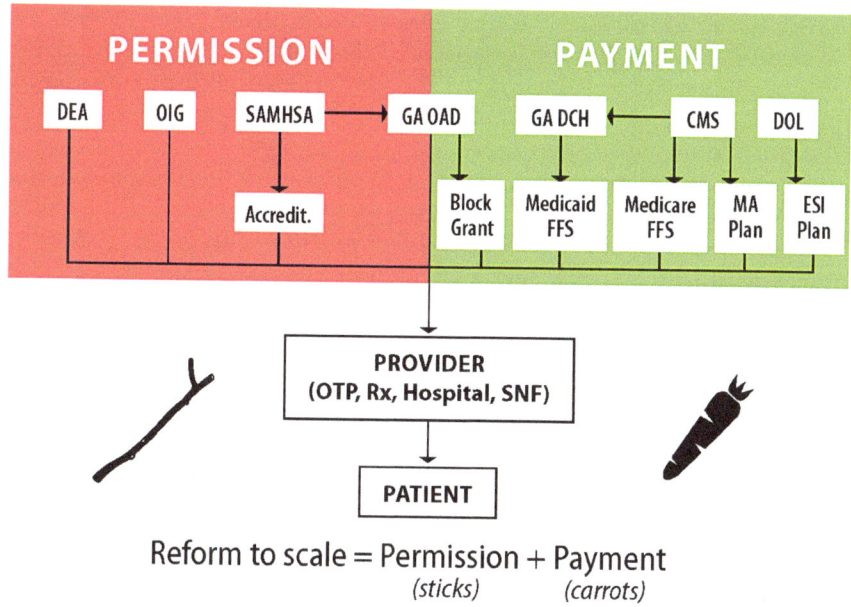

FIGURE 8-2 A simplified illustration of the regulatory environment for provision of methadone. The regulatory environment for the provision of methadone consists of sticks and carrots. The sticks are requirements a provider must meet to get permission to provide methadone; carrots are the payments and reimbursements from federal agencies such as CMS or from charitable organizations that are required to maintain and expand operations and provide methadone to patients in need.
NOTE: CMS = Centers for Medicare & Medicaid Services; DEA = Drug Enforcement Administration; DCH = Department of Community Health; DOL = Department of Labor; ESI = employer-sponsored insurance; FFS = fee-for-services; GA = Georgia; MA = Medicare Advantage; OAD = Office of Addictive Diseases; OIG = Office of Inspector General, U.S. Department of Health and Human Services; OTP = opioid treatment program; SAMHSA = Substance Abuse and Mental Health Services Administration; SNF = skilled nursing facility.
SOURCE: Presented by Matthew Lawrence, March 4, 2022.

On the carrots side is a fragmented payment system, with different payers having different coverage requirements, said Lawrence. For example, traditional Medicare provides a payment bundle to OTPs for methadone. "The payment formula for that is threatening to cut rates for OTPs. CMS is considering ways to avoid those cuts, or maybe increase the generosity now, and that is an important source of flexibility that can really matter," he said. There is currently no reimbursement model (e.g., as through Medicare Part D) for non-OTP options, but Lawrence suggested that the Centers for Medicare & Medicaid Services (CMS) could create more flexible reimbursement options.

Medicare Advantage plans, or "privatized Medicare" as Lawrence put it, employs use management approaches, which often include prior authorization, copays, and step therapy to determine coverage. Whether these plans provide adequate coverage for methadone treatment is unclear, he said. "We just don't know what's happening in that black box."

Lawrence noted that the Center for Medicare and Medicaid Innovation (CMMI) has broad authority to test different payment models and roll them out nationwide if they are successful. For example, they tested a diabetes prevention program in a few geographic areas and found it successful before rolling it out. "That's kind of a wide-open lane to test experiments with improving access to methadone," said Lawrence.

Medicaid managed care is also a black box, said Lawrence. But he noted that Medicaid has broad authority to increase payments to states through section 1115 waivers and could exercise that authority to promote access to methadone through state Medicaid programs, also potentially wrapping in housing, transportation, and other services.

Employer-sponsored insurance plans are required by federal law—the Mental Health Parity and Addiction Equity Act of 2008 and amendments to the Affordable Care Act—to provide benefits for mental health or substance use disorder that are similar to medical and surgical benefits. However, Lawrence said enforcement of this law by the Department of Labor has been limited and there are reports of employer group plans wrongly denying coverage for methadone.

Given that these regulatory pathways exist to expand flexibilities for take-homes and telehealth, Lawrence asked why it took a global pandemic to implement changes. Racism and stigma may be partially responsible, but he suggested that another important factor is ossification. The high costs of regulatory change create a strong bias for maintaining the status quo, even when everyone agrees it is not working, he said. In terms of the regulatory environment for methadone, Lawrence identified several contributors to ossification: (1) horizontal fragmentation among different agencies within the federal government with authority over methadone regulation; (2) extensive vertical fragmentation from federal and state agencies as well as institutional players and individual providers; (3) an organized expert industry in the form of OTPs that are constituents of this regulatory environment; and (4) disempowered regulatory beneficiaries—patients and potential patients who are inherently disempowered as a result of their disease as well as other marginalizing factors.

Lawrence outlined potential solutions to each of these contributors to ossification:

- To address horizontal fragmentation, what is needed, he said, is energetic executive leadership through HHS or the Office of

National Drug Control Policy (ONDCP) with agenda-setting authority, which could launch a methadone "moonshot" similar to President Biden's cancer moonshot. Horizontal fragmentation could also be simplified by pooling authorities, said Lawrence.
- Vertical fragmentation might be addressed by having federal authorities encourage state alignment, for example, by having CMS issue a guidance and invite states to apply for waivers to test different models for providing methadone to patients.
- To empower regulatory beneficiaries, Lawrence said options are available to expand petitions for rulemaking that allow beneficiaries to be the ones who set the agendas for consideration of regulatory changes. He also suggested that agencies could better publicize and respond to complaints from patients.

BOX 8-1
Suggested Regulatory Changes to Remove Barriers to and Incentivize Expanded Methadone Access Proposed by Individual Workshop Participants

- Providing greater flexibility in current regulations by using DEA's authority (21 CFR 1307.03) to grant exceptions to many methadone regulations and SAMHSA's similar authority (42 CFR 8.11(h)) with regard to OTP regulations (C. Davis).
- Revising take-home guidelines so that take-home doses are the default, rather than the exception, and allow flexibility in the initial dose (C. Davis).
- Eliminate the limitation that methadone for OUD only be available at OTPs (C. Davis).
- Revising regulations to permit OTPs to initiate methadone treatment via telemedicine (C. Davis).
- Modifying Medicare/Medicaid regulations and incentives to encourage states to enact state laws that are no more restrictive than federal law and increase the generosity of federal Medicaid payments to states (C. Davis, Lawrence).
- Requiring Medicare-funded resident physicians to receive training in opioid use disorder diagnosis and treatment (C. Davis).
- Conditioning Medicare funding on hospitals providing medications for opioid use disorder in the emergency department and elsewhere (C. Davis).
- Creating alternative, unbundled Medicare and Medicaid payment models that enable reimbursement for pharmacy and non-OTP physician dispensing of methadone, and funding for supports such as housing and transportation (C. Davis, Lawrence).
- Simplifying horizontal fragmentation by pooling authorities (e.g., the Drug Enforcement Administration could deputize the Center for Medicare and Medicaid Innovation by waiving all providers participating in payment model tests or consider nationwide payment model expansions) (Lawrence).
- Using federal authorities to encourage state alignment (Lawrence).
- Including perspectives of people with lived experience receiving or being unable to access methadone treatment in agenda setting (Lawrence).

NOTE: This list is the rapporteurs' summary of points made by the individual speakers identified, and the statements have not been endorsed or verified by the National Academies of Sciences, Engineering, and Medicine. They are not intended to reflect a consensus among workshop participants.

9

Frameworks to Guide the Assessment of Legal and Regulatory Challenges

> **HIGHLIGHTS**
> - Current policies regarding the supply and delivery of methadone have resulted in low treatment rates overall as well as inequities across different population groups (R. Frank).
> - Potential alternatives to current policies include changes to where methadone can be prescribed and dispensed and under what type of supervision, and changes to reimbursement guidelines (R. Frank).
> - Projected outcomes of potential policy changes can be assessed experimentally or by studying "natural experiments" (R. Frank).
> - A policy analysis framework requires making value judgments and weighting outcomes, projecting policy impacts of different alternatives, and considering feasibility and the likely challenges to implementation such as political and community support (R. Frank).
> - Communicating the findings of a policy analysis to a wide range of stakeholders is the most important step toward making meaningful change (R. Frank).
> - To conduct an economic evaluation of potential policy changes, economists perform cost analysis, cost-offset analysis, cost-effectiveness analysis, cost-utility analysis, and benefit–cost analysis, which inform policy makers of the true comprehensive "costs" of a policy (French).

- "Hidden costs" such as travel time can make even a "free" treatment too costly for patients (French).
- Downstream cost savings, for example, from harm reduction programs, may be significant for society, although the savings may not be realized by the agency that incurs the costs (French).
- Cost-utility analysis assesses cost effectiveness, taking into account improvements in quality and duration of life, but may not adequately capture other benefits of addiction treatment (French).

NOTE: This list is the rapporteurs' summary of points made by the individual speakers identified, and the statements have not been endorsed or verified by the National Academies of Sciences, Engineering, and Medicine. They are not intended to reflect a consensus among workshop participants.

The opioid epidemic claimed more than 100,000 American lives in 2021, said Richard Frank, the Margaret T. Morris professor of health economics emeritus at Harvard Medical School and Senior Fellow at the Brookings Institution. Only about 20 percent of the people who need care receive it, and of those only about one-third receive evidence-based treatment. Expanding the use of opioid agonist treatment is a priority as a response to the epidemic, said Frank. Achieving this will require analysis and revision of policies and regulations as well as economic evaluation of potential policy changes.

A POLICY ANALYSIS FRAMEWORK TO SUPPORT HEALTH POLICY DECISIONS

To facilitate workshop discussions on how best to identify policy measures that would most effectively expand the use of methadone, Frank proposed a seven-step policy analysis framework, focusing this framework on regulations that affect the supply of methadone and accompanying policies that might be changed to improve health and well-being by reducing harms associated with opioid use disorder (OUD).

Step 1. Define the policy problem. As the first step in his policy analysis, Frank defined the problem as policies that have resulted in unacceptably low treatment rates, unmet needs, and access challenges for certain population segments, such as racial and ethnic minorities, LGBTQIA+ persons, and rural populations. Contributors to these treatment access problems are the settings where policies will apply, including prisons and jails, local health and human services infrastructures, communities, and different types of housing and living arrangements. Characterizing these different components with data is necessary to understand the heterogeneity of the populations for which policy alternatives will be designed, he said.

Step 2. Set out the policy alternative. Some of the alternatives proposed by individuals throughout the workshop include expanding organizational settings where methadone can be prescribed and dispensed, changing supervision administration rules, and altering insurance coverage and payment policies, said Frank. He noted that specific policy alternatives vary by setting and population segment. For example, the interaction of Medicaid and prison policy is a classic case of how a large national payment policy structure interacts with a particular context and specific setting, he said.

Frank suggested that the policy alternatives most likely to succeed are bundles of complementary policies designed specifically to address desired outcomes, but with appropriate attention to potential unintended consequences, implementation uncertainty, and potential community resistance. "Too often we try to effect change by changing one important policy element, and then are frequently disappointed when the desired outcomes are not realized …. Creating policies that can be dialed up or down is critically important," he said, so that policy makers can make corrections if needed. With regard to methadone treatment, such flexible policies could also enable providers to tailor delivery of take-homes, for example, in order to mitigate harms or anticipated harms, he said.

Step 3. Assemble the relevant evidence. The third step, said Frank, is to assemble evidence that will inform tradeoffs among alternatives. This may involve conducting experiments or studying natural experiments to see, for example, how allowing pharmacists to dispense methadone works, or analyzing how changes in Medicaid coverage or payment policies might affect methadone use and health impacts. During this evidence-collecting period, Frank said it is also important to consider how likely it is that a policy will be implemented as designed or how it might veer away from the original design; how different stakeholders are likely to respond to various policy alternatives; and what the potential is for unintended consequences. He added that outcome projections should include reporting on the sensitivity of outcomes to modest changes in assumptions or altered circumstances.

Step 4. Set out value judgments that underpin the choice of best alternatives. The fourth step in Frank's policy framework requires making value judgments about how to weigh outcomes when tradeoffs need to be made.

Step 5. Project the policy impacts of different alternatives.

Step 6. Consider the tradeoffs. Frank said this is the most difficult. It requires putting together all the evidence about how the various alternatives will work with respect to impacts, implementation, feasibility, political acceptability, and community support. For example, if a policy is designed to expand access and continuation in treatment, one must consider the likelihood that those benefits will be realized, the risks of negative outcomes in certain communities and the tolerance of those communities for the risk, and the costs of one alternative compared to others.

Step 7. Build a narrative. Frank said the last and most important feature of this policy analysis is building a narrative and communicating with a wide range of stakeholders about what has been learned through the process. He noted that conducting this policy analysis will not be easy, in light of the limited evidence available on different approaches to methadone in the United States. "We have very few data points on [which] to build an evidentiary basis for playing with different types of policy designs in building up the alternatives and bringing evidence to them," said Frank, noting however that pandemic regulatory relief offers some opportunities to begin building a U.S.-specific evidentiary foundation. For example, evidence now exists regarding the consequences of expanding Medicaid generally and specifically for addiction treatment, yet there is far less data concerning other regulatory provisions, such as changing Medicaid rules for incarcerated populations, he said.

Creating policies that make meaningful change in the capacity to address medications for OUD requires policy makers to understand all the different levers that need to be pulled rather than looking at each policy in isolation, said Frank. This includes economic levers, he said, "and there are probably five or six hidden levers inside that." For example, building capacity to treat people with methadone may require going beyond asking the federal government to invest in solutions. Rather, he said, a combination of federal and market investments may be needed. Venture capital is one potential resource, but raises concerns about whether those resources will be deployed in a way that maximizes social benefits in an equitable way. "You need to anticipate those unwanted responses and create regulations, accountability, and metrics so that you can monitor and manage those issues," said Frank.

A COST-EFFECTIVENESS FRAMEWORK TO ASSESS POTENTIAL LEGAL AND REGULATORY CHANGES

Economic evaluation of addiction treatment is a relatively recent practice, in part because some of the techniques used for evaluating traditional physical health care interventions do not translate well to addiction programs, which are concerned not just with the patient, but with society as well, said Michael French, professor and chair of the department of health management and policy at the Miami Herbert Business School, University of Miami. He added that economic evaluation provides just one data point that, along with clinical and programmatic evaluations, goes into a policy maker's decision-making process.

Like Frank, French presented a framework for conducting an economic evaluation rather than results from specific studies. A cost analysis is nearly always the first step, he said, adding that economists think about costs not just in terms of dollars, but also in terms of the value of various resources. Hidden costs, such as patient travel time and the costs associated with program volunteers and overhead resources, are also important to include, said French. These hidden costs can make even "free" treatment too costly for patients. To aid in the collection of information on resources used in delivery of treatment for substance use disorder, French and colleagues developed an instrument called DATCAP—the Drug Abuse Treatment Cost Analysis Program.[1]

Another type of evaluation that helps determine if investing in a certain resource or treatment will lead to cost savings down the road is called cost-offset analysis, said French. This type of analysis is particularly useful for harm reduction programs, he said. For example, investing in needle exchange programs can help avoid future costs in terms of hepatitis C infection, HIV, and overdoses.

A challenge in this regard is that the agencies that deal with health and those that deal with crime are not connected and may have very different priorities, said French. For example, when he and his colleagues conduct treatment evaluations in criminal justice settings, they provide a full and comprehensive examination of outcomes, including societal outcomes. However, the interest of the correctional facility may be limited to the cost of delivering treatment in prison and, perhaps, recidivism. That is a very narrow perspective, which ignores potential benefits beyond just not committing crimes, said French. His solution is to present a narrow perspective to the agency sponsoring the research, and then augmenting that with a societal analysis for people and agencies interested in ancillary outcomes.

Cost-effectiveness analysis is used to assess the incremental cost of an intervention compared to something else, which could be an alternative intervention, usual treatment, or even doing nothing, said French. He added that if doing nothing leads to an outcome, however modest, that also needs to be subtracted from the outcome of the interventions. Some of the possible outcomes that could be assessed for the two alternatives include number of drug-using days, success in obtaining employment, and arrests, among others, said French. A challenge with conducting a cost-effectiveness analysis in this area is the lack of consistent benchmarks for acceptable

---

[1] To learn more about DATCAP, go to https://datcap.com (accessed April 20, 2022).

costs for achieving a certain outcome. For example, said French, "If I said to you that an intervention achieved a drug-free week at a cost of $50, most people would say that seems pretty reasonable. But if was $500 or $5,000, now a debate starts."

Another limitation of cost-effectiveness analysis is that it can only examine one outcome at a time, which does not fit well with addiction interventions because the outcomes are multidimensional, spanning both individual and societal issues, he said. Economists call these externalities, said French. For example, substance use can lead an individual to commit crimes to pay for the drugs, or it can cause family discord, job loss, or educational disruption, all of which can be considered costs.

A third challenge with regard to cost-effectiveness analysis, said French, is that while economists have various ways of incorporating uncertainty into their analyses to come up with estimates that are somewhat imprecise with big confidence intervals, decision makers want very specific point estimates.

French said the most common economic analysis approach used in the medical literature is cost-utility analysis, which is an extension of-cost effectiveness analysis, but with an outcome that takes into account improvements in both the quality and duration of life, such as quality-adjusted life years. Like cost-effectiveness analysis, cost-utility analysis does not adequately capture the benefits of addiction treatment beyond patient well-being and duration of life.

A final economic analysis approach is called benefit–cost analysis, which incorporates all the outcomes that are applicable to an addiction intervention, said French. It is much more comprehensive, complicated, and costly, but provides policy makers with information that is easily understood and makes dollar-to-dollar comparisons, he said. For example, if a program has a benefit–cost ratio of four to one, it is returning $4 for every $1 invested, said French. The results of this analysis can also be reported as net benefits, namely, the total benefit minus the total cost.

The advantage of economic analysis, according to French, is rather than saying a treatment works—which could mean that it works sometimes, but not always—this analysis quantifies the benefit of a treatment in comparison to other alternatives. He listed several recommendations for researchers considering an economic evaluation:

- Develop a concise research question or hypothesis.
- Recruit a team of researchers that can initiate the economic analysis at the beginning of your project.
- Define every alternative program or intervention.

- Clearly define the perspective of the analysis (e.g., patient, society, taxpayers, treatment facility, insurance company, criminal justice agency, etc.).
- Include all externalities, pain and suffering, shared resources, and hidden costs.
- Assess the generalizability of the study findings.
- Base your decisions on marginal (i.e., the cost to produce one additional service or product) rather than average costs and benefits.

10

Moving Forward: Potential Concrete Legal and Regulatory Actions

HIGHLIGHTS

- Including the perspectives of people taking methadone and others who use drugs in policy reforms is essential (D. Frank, Rucker, Weizman).
- "Success" in methadone treatment needs to be redefined to include non-abstinence-based recovery and pain relief (Brooklyn, D. Frank, Rucker).
- A less restrictive and more patient-oriented approach to the treatment of opioid use disorder (OUD) is needed (Bonnie).
- Federal agencies have authority to take actions most urgently needed (Bonnie, C. Davis, Dooling, Lawrence, Weizman).
- A bold, clear, long-term strategic vision is needed to reform the opioid treatment program (OTP) system and provide universal access to methadone for OUD (Weizman).
- Reforms most urgently needed include: extending take-home flexibilities, addressing coverage barriers, incentivizing states to expand methadone access, increasing flexibility at OTPs in prescribing and dispensing medications for OUD, allowing greater room for clinical discretion, and providing Americans with Disabilities Act enforcement guidance (Bonnie).
- Incentives to states and providers will be needed to ensure implementation of any new paradigm (Weizman).

- States have the ability to extend COVID-19 flexibilities, as demonstrated in New York (Cunningham).
- Applying to correctional facilities the framework used in hospitals to provide methadone would improve treatment of a population at very high risk (Saloner).
- Tethering access to federal funds to a restriction against using methadone as grounds for family separation could help reduce the number of children going into foster care (Weizman).
- Modernizing the collection of data related to methadone treatment could increase understanding of the current status of methadone access and quality of care for methadone patients (Saloner).
- Fully integrating opioid treatment into the health care system would improve care and outcomes by ensuring cross-disciplinary collaboration and peer review (Brooklyn).

NOTE: This list is the rapporteurs' summary of points made by the individual speakers identified, and the statements have not been endorsed or verified by the National Academies of Sciences, Engineering, and Medicine. They are not intended to reflect a consensus among workshop participants.

The final session of the workshop aimed to review the presentations and discussions regarding potential legal and regulatory changes, as well as to seek reflections from people with a broad range of perspectives on the workshop discussions within a broader context of reforming drug policy and treatment for opioid use disorder (OUD).

LEGAL AND REGULATORY REFORMS

"For far too long, policy discourse on addiction has largely been directed to mediating conflict rather than developing and effectuating a consensus," said Richard Bonnie, the Harrison Foundation professor of medicine and law and director of the Institute of Law, Psychiatry, and Public Policy at the University of Virginia. However, he said, presentations and discussions over the course of this workshop reflect a common understanding of the nature of addiction and the therapeutic benefits of methadone and reflect "support of a less restrictive and more patient-oriented approach to the treatment of opioid use disorder and the use of medications for opioid use disorder." Moreover, he said, several workshop participants with legal expertise participating in the workshop noted "that the relevant federal agencies already currently have ample legal authority" to take the actions that are most urgently needed to facilitate a more effective and patient-centered approach to the use of medication for OUD in general, and to methadone in particular.

Bonnie summarized six points discussed by several workshop participants with legal expertise (Bridget Dooling, Corey Davis, Matthew Lawrence, and Shelly Weizman, associate director of the Addiction and Public Policy Initiative at the O'Neill Institute for National and Global Health Law, Georgetown University Law Center), which were subsequently published after the meeting (Bonnie et al., 2022).[1]

Extending "take-home" flexibilities. In response to the COVID-19 public health emergency, the Substance Abuse and Mental Health Services Administration (SAMHSA) agreed to extend methadone take-home flexibilities for 1 year after the COVID-19 public health emergency expires while working on a permanent solution, said Bonnie. However, he noted that rulemaking is a time-consuming process that can become delayed or derailed during administrative transitions. "Our legal experts were of one mind in urging SAMHSA to couple its planned rulemaking with expeditious action to reauthorize current take-home flexibilities under the existing 'opioid crisis' public health emergency," he said, assuming that a permanent solution will be much more flexible in allowing take-home access.

Using authority over public programs to check coverage barriers imposed by insurers. As was discussed by several participants during this workshop, insurer policies may interfere with patient–doctor relationships in employer-sponsored insurance, Medicaid managed care, and Medicare Advantage. Congress is currently considering parity reform legislation, which would give the Department of Labor more authority in relation to employer-sponsored insurance, said Bonnie, adding the Centers for Medicare & Medicaid Services (CMS) could do much to address insurance barriers in public programs. In particular, Bonnie said, "CMS should consider OTP [opioid treatment program] coverage in assessing Medicare Advantage network adequacy; should reevaluate and strengthen its risk adjustment model's application to substance use disorders; and should collect and scrutinize data on barriers in Medicaid managed care. CMS has the authority to do all these things," he said (Bonnie et al., 2022); CMS can also offer states a specific Medicaid demonstration opportunity to expand access to methadone under its section 1115 waiver authority. Such an initiative should prioritize access, quality, and integration into a state's existing continuum of health and social services, said Bonnie.

Using existing federal authorities to incentivize states to enable expanded methadone access. One problem that was discussed in some detail is state policies relating to methadone access that are more restrictive than the federal policy, said Bonnie. This is a serious problem, he said; however, the federal government has tremendous leveraging tools at its disposal in

---

[1] They are not meant to be viewed as formal recommendations of the National Academies.

situations of this kind. Specifically, it can tether certain incentives to block grants and other grant programs when state policies are more restrictive than the federal policy or when federal agencies want to incentivize states to undertake innovations. Bonnie suggested that this leveraging authority should be used more aggressively to "incentivize states to implement new models designed to expand methadone access, including in different populations (e.g., pregnant and parenting) and settings (e.g., prisons, jails, long-term care facilities, and inpatient substance use disorder treatment facilities)." He added that "federal agencies can also offer targeted technical assistance to states and providers to: 1) operationalize changes in the federal methadone regulatory framework, 2) implement federal parity rules, 3) adjust Medicaid reimbursement structures to align with best practices for care, and 4) rapidly translate new research into policy and practice" (Bonnie et al., 2022).

Using existing rulemaking authority to provide greater flexibility in the current regulations governing prescribing, dispensing, and treatment by OTPs. SAMHSA and the Drug Enforcement Administration (DEA) have the authority to mend most, if not all, of the regulations restricting methadone dispensing and prescribing by OTPs that critics of the existing regulations have proposed, said Bonnie. Examples include relaxing take-home limitations, dosing requirements on methadone, and toxicology screening requirements.

Using existing rulemaking authority to allow greater room for clinical discretion. The regulatory presumption should favor informed clinical judgment and respect the traditional orientation of the patient–clinician relationship, said Bonnie. Provisions that he suggested merit reconsideration include:

- Eliminating daily dose requirements.
- Expanding authority for otherwise authorized and registered prescribers to outside of OTPs. This can include expanding the types of facilities and programs that can provide treatment using methadone, including primary care, Federally Qualified Health Centers (FQHCs), certified community behavioral health clinics, mobile units, and harm reduction facilities.
- Eliminating mandatory eight-times-a-year toxicology screens.
- Updating criteria for take-home doses to meet patient needs and defer to the treating clinician.
- Allowing patients to access methadone at a pharmacy.
- Developing a specific regulatory framework for methadone in carceral settings with the goal of facilitating access.

Providing enforcement guidance on obligations imposed by the Americans with Disabilities Act (ADA) with particular attention to facilitating access to methadone in prisons and jails. Bonnie and colleagues added that methadone patients' civil rights should be a top enforcement priority among relevant federal agencies, including the Department of Justice's Office of Civil Rights, U.S. Attorneys' Offices, and the Department of Health and Human Services' (HHS's) Office of Civil Rights. Enforcement guidance is needed to explain the full extent of protections under the ADA[2] and other applicable laws. Bonnie added that prisons, providers, or other entities found to be in violation of these laws should be investigated immediately.

EXPLORING OPPORTUNITIES TO REFORM METHADONE TREATMENT

Reform has to start with a bold, clear, and long-term strategic vision, said Weizman—perhaps a "methadone moonshot," such as that suggested by Lawrence. Improving the system as it is now should be pursued in parallel with working toward long-term reform with intentional goals and sustained investment, she said, noting that this vision is in line with President Biden's goal of universal access to medications for OUD by 2025, which he embraced in his State of the Union address.

A critical reform, according to Weizman, is a reconceptualization of OTPs. Even with incremental improvements, she said, an insufficient number of OTPs exist to meet the needs of patients. Different models and new paradigms for delivery of methadone are needed, which could include a range of solutions discussed at this workshop: a hub-and-spoke model, with OTPs, FQHCs, and/or community behavioral health centers serving as hubs; and pharmacies, hospitals, primary care providers, correctional facilities, or other providers serving as spokes where patients can receive care and treatment.

Alternatively, said Weizman, the buprenorphine model of prescribing and delivering medication could be adopted for methadone. "Whatever model is selected, it has to be part of a cohesive vision not only for methadone, but also for how we address addiction generally."

Any new paradigm must be incentivized and supported by states and providers, using the many tools provided by the federal government, said Weizman. She suggested that Medicaid could facilitate reform by offering state Medicaid demonstration opportunities, waiver services, and alternative reimbursement structures. States and providers will need guidance on how to maximize these opportunities, she added; the entire system will need a deep commitment to technical assistance and financial support. Weizman also advocated tethering access to federal funds to a requirement that states

---

[2] Following this workshop, the U.S. Department of Justice issued guidance on protections under the American with Disabilities Act. To learn more, go to https://www.ada.gov/opioid_guidance.pdf (accessed June 12, 2022).

cannot use methadone as grounds for removal of children, termination of parental rights, or engagement of child protective services.

Underscoring the importance of regulatory reform for methadone in correctional facilities, Brendan Saloner, Bloomberg Associate Professor of American health and addiction and overdose at Johns Hopkins School of Public Health, noted that the Medicaid Reentry Act would provide funding to provide treatment for people in prisons as well as a bridge back to the community, but as part of President Biden's Build Back Better framework, faces an uncertain future in Congress.

To get started on these reforms, Weizman urged (1) retaining COVID-19 flexibilities; (2) moving from a legal framework guided by rigid regulations to a clinical approach (e.g., starting with daily dose and counseling requirements); and (3) expanding the authority for otherwise authorized and registered prescribers to dispense at remote locations. She advocated prioritizing high-risk populations, such as people in corrections and pregnant and postpartum women.

Weizman added that a bridge is needed to nimbly connect research to policy, which again will require technical assistance. For example, she noted that there has been substantial research on the consequences of the COVID-19 regulatory flexibilities, targeted research on the best way to approach illicitly manufactured fentanyl, and research on population-specific best practices.

REFORMING METHADONE TREATMENT WITHIN THE BROADER CONTEXT FOR IMPROVING ACCESS TO MEDICATIONS FOR OPIOID USE DISORDER

Individual workshop participants discussed several concrete next steps that could improve access to methadone, but would not require regulatory changes or new legislation. Weizman emphasized that implementation will require using a combination of different policy and legal tools. Some states and local governments are ready, but others will need to be pushed, she said. It is not done simply through the stroke of a pen, she said. "I think it's a matter of the right combination of carrots and sticks and incentives and mandates that is going to get it done."

Incorporating All Voices at Every Stage of the Reform Process

Any reforms under consideration should incorporate at every step of the way the perspective of people with OUD and those receiving methadone, including people with long histories in the system, activists, and even people who use drugs but are not in treatment, said Weizman. Joy Rucker, co-founder and former executive director of the Texas Harm Reduction

Alliance, agreed, saying she supported having people from the Urban Survivor's Union,[3] a grassroots organization of people who use drugs, participate in decision making about how methadone should be distributed. She referred to the organization's *Methadone Manifesto* that was co-authored by people with lived experience. "The best way to create a system and make a policy change is to have the people that are most impacted and affected by these policies relate to you exactly what the impact of the policies [is] on their day-to-day lives," said Rucker.

Redefining Success in Methadone Treatment

As a person who has been on methadone maintenance for nearly 20 years, David Frank, medical sociologist at the New York University School of Global Public Health, has a unique perspective on the disconnect between the way methadone is administered and how it is actually used. Methadone enabled Frank to get a bank account, maintain a job, and eventually to earn a Ph.D., yet while he appears to be one of methadone's great success stories, he said he is not pursuing abstinence-based recovery and has never been compliant with the rules of his clinic. He suggested that success in methadone treatment needs to be redefined, and policies reconsidered to enable non-abstinence-based recovery.

Frank said he started using methadone as a way to continue using opioids, but avoid the difficulties and risks associated with criminalized opioid use. He said he continues to use drugs, including heroin, although less often and in a safer way than before he started methadone maintenance. But to do this, he said, "I have had to lie to counselors and doctors, restrict where I live to places that have access to clinics that aren't testing for particular substances, and occasionally even fake drug tests." Had he not employed these tactics, he said, he would have been forced out of treatment; he would have never been able to get his Ph.D. or begun working in the field if he was required to go to a clinic every single morning.

Frank noted that many people benefit tremendously from methadone, but are not interested in becoming abstinent. In a recent study, he found that while some people want to achieve abstinence, many people were more interested in stability and getting out of a chaotic lifestyle than in abstinence. Some wanted to continue using heroin or other drugs, but wanted to make sure they were never in withdrawal (Frank and Walters, 2021). He mentioned one person he spoke to as part of his dissertation who had completely stopped using heroin, but was required to come to the clinic every day because he continued to smoke marijuana and use alcohol. Frustrated

---

[3] For more information on the Urban Survivor's Union, go to https://ncurbansurvivorunion.org/national-usu (accessed May 4, 2022).

with this requirement and unhappy with the treatment he received at the clinic, he quit and died of a fentanyl overdose shortly thereafter.

Frank advocated moving away from the punitive focus on abstinence and embrace policies that enable people who continue to use drugs to stay in methadone and receive take-home doses, as they often are allowed with buprenorphine. John Brooklyn, clinical associate professor of family medicine and psychiatry at the University of Vermont (UVM) Larner College of Medicine and a physician expert in the UVM Center on Rural Addiction, added that as someone who treats thousands of people with methadone, his first question as a doctor is "what is your goal?" For some it is relief from pain, he said, while others wish to reduce their use or achieve abstinence. The goal may change over time, he said, but the policy of the program may not align with the patient's wishes. If a program works with the patient, meets them where they are, and takes their goals as well as safety into consideration, Brooklyn believes people can be very successful.

Rucker echoed Frank's and Brooklyn's comments, adding, "We need to let people define what their recovery looks like." Rucker also has lived experience with methadone as well as with suboxone and abstinence. The stigma associated with methadone use can be crippling and could be addressed by allowing people to pick up their medication in pharmacies rather than standing in line at a methadone clinic, she said. She recalled traveling long distances to a methadone clinic far from her home or work simply so she could have some anonymity. Rucker also opposed mandatory counseling and advocated delivery of opioid treatment to incarcerated people as well as continuation of that treatment upon release.

"Methadone has been used as a social control mechanism throughout the years and that is why we have all these barriers to access," she said. "That is what needs to change." Frank agreed, adding that the criminalization of methadone maintenance should be viewed in the context of the war on drugs and prohibition.

Providing Methadone through a Hub-and-Spoke Model

Vermont has established opioid treatment programs using a hub-and-spoke model, said Brooklyn. The hubs are centers of excellence located throughout the state that provide high-intensity, medication-assisted treatment connected to spokes in the community, which provide maintenance medication assisted treatment and other services, said Brooklyn. He said the hubs also have robust transfers back and forth from inpatient, residential situations, obstetricians, and the criminal justice system.

One of the challenges in Vermont and elsewhere in the United States is providing methadone to rural communities, said Brooklyn. He initiated a project where patients were given a secure medication dispenser and a video app that enabled them to record themselves taking their medication, with the videos time and date stamped. This video-direct observed therapy approach has been used successfully for patients with tuberculosis, he said.

The project enrolled 58 patients, 41 of them on methadone and 17 on buprenorphine. Brooklyn said at the start of the project, 83 percent of the people in the study did not meet take-home criteria. Of the 15,581 videos received, only one showed evidence of diversion, he said. After 1 year, 98 percent of the participants were still in treatment, prosocial activities had increased from 79 percent to 93 percent, and patients reported weekly travel time savings of 5.5 hours and weekly travel cost savings of $72.00.

The Vermont program addresses both providers' fears about diversion, drug use, and induction safety, while also addressing patients' fears about missing work, clinic, or school, their lack of transportation, and concerns about stigma, said Brooklyn. He suggested that this model could be extended to rural communities throughout the United States. However, several workshop participants with lived experience expressed deep concerns about the use of video-direct observed therapy.

Integrating Opioid Treatment Fully into the Medical System

In other fields of medicine, providers and researchers work collaboratively and there is constant peer review, said Brooklyn. OTPs, in contrast, operate as fiefdoms and there is little peer oversight, he said. Perhaps, said Brooklyn, opioid treatment should be integrated fully into the medical system so that there is collaboration across disciplines, rather than living in a siloed world where the treatment received depends on the clinic administering the treatment. With national standards, such as those that exist for the treatment of diabetes or cancer, peer review could help mitigate poor treatment, he said. "Methadone programs should provide a full range of services; and if they can't, they should be integrated into other areas that can help people become healthy humans and not just be patients on methadone," said Brooklyn.

A Comprehensive Statewide Approach

The state of New York, which has more than 96 OTPs serving 40,000 patients, has already begun efforts to extend COVID-19 flexibilities, said Chinazo Cunningham, commissioner of the New York State Office of Addiction Services and Supports. Funding for 35 mobile methadone units linked to brick-and-mortar OTPs is planned, she said. They are also encouraging the use of telehealth and expanding a methadone delivery program started during the pandemic. To further improve access, they have added bundled payment rates to existing ambulatory patient group rates that they hope will reduce the number of visits required for medication administration by paying programs for their services by the week regardless of whether a patient comes in for medication administration.

To reach one of the highest risk populations—people who are incarcerated in correctional facilities—New York Governor Hochul signed a law mandating that all jails and prisons across the state offer all three approved medications for opioid use disorder. Implementing the law will be challenging and will require funding from the state or opioid settlement money or other sources to enable implementation, said Cunningham. She added that they are also hoping to change the ability of skilled nursing facilities, residential treatment programs, and long-term care facilities to store and administer methadone.

Cunningham said her agency is also starting a harm reduction division to look at how treatment is implemented. "We need to focus on keeping people alive," she said.

Modernizing the Data Collection Process

Alongside regulatory changes needed across the methadone treatment landscape, Saloner also emphasized the need to modernize the data collection process. "There are huge holes in our understanding of access and quality of care for methadone patients," he said, as well as a lack of answers to fundamental questions such as how many people want access but cannot get it, how many new patients begin methadone treatment each year, and what the rates of retention are.

Saloner listed four elements of a modernized data strategy:

- Improving the National Survey of Drug Use and Health, which although it now collects data on use of methadone, misses critical populations as it does not reach into correctional facilities or interview people experiencing homelessness.
- Collecting methadone treatment use data as part of the national Treatment Episode Data Set (TEDS).[4]
- Undertaking a national longitudinal cohort study of methadone patients to better understand factors related to recovery outcomes and retention in treatment.
- Planning for data collection outside of OTPs, for example, at mobile units, long-term care facilities, office-based settings, pharmacies, and, as mentioned above, correctional facilities.

---

[4] To learn more about TEDS, go to https://www.samhsa.gov/data/data-we-collect/teds-treatment-episode-data-set#teds_a (accessed May 4, 2022).

Understanding the Real-World Impact of Policy Interventions

While many studies have shown that methadone is effective, there is less known about how a changing policy environment would affect real-world populations, said Saloner. "We need to have a subtle and nuanced understanding of how specific policy interventions are saving lives and having an impact on other kinds of socially important metrics."

CLOSING REMARKS

"We have got the momentum going for policy change," said Bonnie. From the bottom up, this will mean formulating not only policy experiments, but also the research that goes along with that. The discussions of this workshop provide a good starting point from which people can be brought together to devise a sensible research strategy. The top-down part, he said, relates to what the Office of National Drug Control Policy (ONDCP) and the White House will do next and how they will leverage their authority to move forward. Alan Leshner concurred, calling this a "landmark moment." "It is the first time we have had ONDCP, SAMHSA, other parts of HHS, and [the] DEA all saying we need to expand access and address disparities."

A

References

Ahmad, F. B., L. M. Rossen, and P. Sutton. 2021 Provisional drug overdose death counts. *Vital Statistics Rapid Release: National Center for Health Statistics.* 2021. https://www.cdc.gov/nchs/nvss/vsrr/drug-overdose-data.htm#citation (accessed June 10, 2022).

Almazan, A. N., D. King, C. Grasso, S. Cahill, M. Lattanner, M. L. Hatzenbuehler, and A. S. Keuroghlian. 2021. Sexual orientation and gender identity data collection at US health centers: Impact of city-level structural stigma in 2018. *American Journal of Public Health* 111(11):2059–2063. https://doi.org/10.2105/AJPH.2021.306414.

APA (American Psychiatric Association). 2022. Diagnostic and statistical manual of mental disorders: DSM-5-TR. Washington, DC: American Psychiatric Association.

Anstice, A., C. J. Strike, and B. Brands. 2009. Supervised methadone consumption: Client issues and stigma, *Substance Use & Misuse* 44(6):794–808. https://doi.org/10.1080/10826080802483936.

Baumgartner, J. C., and D. C. Radley. 2022. Overdose deaths surged in the first half of 2021, underscoring urgent need for action. *The Commonwealth Fund.* https://doi.org/10.26099/TMAE-JE82 (accessed April 26, 2022).

Bellamy, C. D., M. Costa, J. Wyatt, M. Mathis, A. Sloan, M. Budge, K. Blackman, L. Ocasio, G. Reis, K. Guy, R. R. Anderson, M. S. Copes, and A. Jordan. 2021. A collaborative culturally-centered and community-driven faith-based opioid recovery initiative: The Imani Breakthrough project. *Social Work in Mental Health* 19(6):558–567. https://doi.org/10.1080/15332985.2021.1930329.

Binswanger, I. A., M. F. Stern, R. A. Deyo, P. J. Heagerty, A. Cheadle, J. G. Elmore, and T. D. Koepsell. 2007. Release from prison—a high risk of death for former inmates. *The New England Journal of Medicine* 356(2):157–165. https://doi.org/10.1056/NEJMsa064115.

Bonnie, R. J., C. Davis, B. C. E. Dooling, M. Lawrence, and S. Weizman. 2022. An expedited regulatory strategy for expanding access to methadone treatment for substance use disorders. *Health Affairs Forefront.* May 27. http://doi.org/10.1377/forefront.20220524.171269.

Bowden, C. L., J. F. Maddux, and M. Esquivel. 1976. Methadone dispensing by community pharmacies. *The American Journal of Drug and Alcohol Abuse* 3(2):243–254. https://doi.org/10.3109/00952997609077194.

Bronson, J., J. Stroop, S. Zimmer, and M. Berzofsky. 2017. Drug use, dependence, and abuse among state prisoners and jail inmates, 2007–2009. *NCJ 250546*. Department of Justice, Bureau of Justice Statistics, Bureau of Justice Statistics. https://bjs.ojp.gov/content/pub/pdf/dudaspji0709.pdf (accessed June 6, 2022).

Brooner, R. K., K. B. Stoller, P. Patel, L. T. Wu, H. Yan, and M. Kidorf. 2022. Opioid treatment program prescribing of methadone with community pharmacy dispensing: Pilot study of feasibility and acceptability. Drug and Alcohol Dependence Reports, p.100067.

Brothers, S., A. Viera, and R. Heimer. 2021. Changes in methadone program practices and fatal methadone overdose rates in Connecticut during COVID-19. *Journal of Substance Abuse Treatment* 131(December):108449. https://doi.org/10.1016/j.jsat.2021.108449.

Bukten, A., M. R. Stavseth, S. Skurtveit, A. Tverdal, J. Strang, and T. Clausen. 2017. High risk of overdose death following release from prison: Variations in mortality during a 15-year observation period. *Addiction* 112(8):1432–1439.

Burns, L., D. Randall, W. D. Hall, M. Law, T. Butler, J. Bell, and L. Degenhardt. 2009. Opioid agonist pharmacotherapy in New South Wales from 1985 to 2006: Patient characteristics and patterns and predictors of treatment retention. *Addiction* 104(8):1363–1372. https://doi.org/10.1111/j.1360-0443.2009.02633.x.

CDC (Centers for Disease Control and Prevention). 2021. *Quarterly provisional drug overdose estimates with demographics (August)*. https://www.cdc.gov/nchs/nvss/vsrr/drug-overdose-data.htm (accessed May 11, 2022).

CDC. 2022. *National Center for Health Statistics: Products–Vital statistics rapid release–Provisional drug overdose data*. https://www.cdc.gov/nchs/nvss/vsrr/drug-overdose-data.htm (accessed April 26, 2022).

Chang, J. E., B. Franz, C. E. Cronin, Z. Lindenfeld, A. Y. Lai, and J. A. Pagán. 2022. Racial/ethnic disparities in the availability of hospital based opioid use disorder treatment. *Journal of Substance Abuse Treatment* February. https://doi.org/10.1016/j.jsat.2022.108719.

Coroners Court of Victoria. 2021. Victorian overdose deaths, 2011–2020. https://www.coronerscourt.vic.gov.au/sites/default/files/2021-07/CCOV%20-%20Overdose%20deaths%20in%20Victoria%202011-2020%20-%2029Jul2021.pdf (accessed June 14, 2022).

Drucker, E., S. Rice, G. Ganse, J. J. Kegley, K. Bonuck, and E. Tuchman. 2007. The Lancaster office based opiate treatment program: A case study and prototype for community physicians and pharmacists providing methadone maintenance treatment in the United States. *Addictive Disorders & Their Treatment* 6:121–135.

Dunn, K. E., R. K. Brooner, K. B. Stoller. 2021. Technology-assisted methadone take-home dosing for dispensing methadone to persons with opioid use disorder during the COVID-19 pandemic. *Journal of Substance Abuse Treatment* 121:108197.

Entress, R. M. 2021. The intersection of race and opioid use disorder treatment: A quantitative analysis. *Journal of Substance Abuse Treatment* 131(December). https://doi.org/10.1016/j.jsat.2021.108589.

Esposito, D., L. Simon, M. Tucker, J. Stangle, T. Moore, I. Hill, B. Courtot, E. Burroughs, and K. Witgert. (2021). Maternal Opioid Misuse (MOM) model: Pre-implementation evaluation report. Centers for Medicare & Medicaid Services. https://innovation.cms.gov/data-and-reports/2022/mom-preimp-report (accessed June 13, 2022).

Fiellin, D. A., P. G. O'Connor, M. Chawarski, J. P. Pakes, M. V. Pantalon, and R. S. Schottenfeld. 2001. Methadone maintenance in primary care: A randomized controlled trial. *Journal of the American Medical Association* 86(14):1724–1731. https://doi.org/10.1001/jama.286.14.1724.

Figgatt, M. C., Z. Salazar, E. Day, L. Vincent, and N. Dasgupta. 2021. Take-home dosing experiences among persons receiving methadone maintenance treatment during COVID-19. *Journal of Substance Abuse Treatment* 123(April):108276. https://doi.org/10.1016/j.jsat.2021.108276.

Fonseca J., and A. Chang, F. Chang. 2018. Perceived barriers and facilitators to providing methadone maintenance treatment among rural community pharmacists in Southwestern Ontario. *Journal of Rural Health* 34(1):23–30. doi:10.1111/jrh.12264.

Frank, D., and S. M. Walters. 2021. 'I'm going to stop myself before someone stops me': Complicating narratives of volitional substance use treatment. *Frontiers in Sociology* 6:619677. https://doi.org/10.3389/fsoc.2021.619677.

Frank, D., P. Mateu-Gelabert, D. C. Perlman, S. M. Walters, L. Curran, and H. Guarino. 2021. "It's like 'liquid handcuffs'": The effects of take-home dosing policies on methadone maintenance treatment (MMT) patients' lives. *Harm Reduction Journal* 18(1):88. https://doi.org/10.1186/s12954-021-00535-y.

Friedman, J., L. Beletsky, and A. Jordan. 2022. Surging racial disparities in the US overdose crisis. *American Journal of Psychiatry* 179(2):166–169. https://doi.org/10.1176/appi.ajp.2021.21040381.

Gauthier, G., J. K. Eibl, and D. C. Marsh. 2018. Improved treatment-retention for patients receiving methadone dosing within the clinic providing physician and other health services (onsite) versus dosing at community (offsite) pharmacies. *Drug and Alcohol Dependence* 191(October):1–5. https://doi.org/10.1016/j.drugalcdep.2018.04.029.

Girouard, M. P., H. Goldhammer, and A. S. Keuroghlian. 2019. Understanding and treating opioid use disorders in lesbian, gay, bisexual, transgender, and queer populations. *Substance Abuse* 40(3):335–339. https://doi.org/10.1080/08897077.2018.1544963.

Goedel, W. C., A. Shapiro, M. Cerdá, J. W. Tsai, S. E. Hadland, and B. D. L. Marshall. 2020. Association of racial/ethnic segregation with treatment capacity for opioid use disorder in counties in the United States. *Journal of American Medicine Association* 3(4):e203711. https://doi.org/10.1001/jamanetworkopen.2020.3711.

Goldhammer, H., A. C. Smart, L. A. Kissock, and A. S. Keuroghlian. 2021. Organizational strategies and inclusive language to build culturally responsive health care environments for lesbian, gay, bisexual, transgender, and queer people. *Journal of Health Care for the Poor and Underserved* 32(1):18–29. https://doi.org/10.1353/hpu.2021.0004.

Hansen, H., C. Siegel, J. Wanderling, and D. DiRocco. 2016. Buprenorphine and methadone treatment for opioid dependence by income, ethnicity and race of neighborhoods in New York City. *Drug and Alcohol Dependence* 164(July):14–21. https://doi.org/10.1016/j.drugalcdep.2016.03.028.

Harris, M. T., A. M. Lambert, A. D. Maschke, S. M. Bagley, A. Y. Walley, and C. M. Gunn. 2021. "No home to take methadone to": Experiences with addiction services during the COVID-19 pandemic among survivors of opioid overdose in Boston. *Journal of Substance Abuse Treatment* 135:108655.

Hatch-Maillette, M. A., K. M. Peavy, J. I. Tsui, C. J. Banta-Green, S. Woolworth, P. Grekin, 2021. Re-thinking patient stability for methadone in opioid treatment programs during a global pandemic: Provider perspectives. *Journal of Substance Abuse Treatment* 124:108223.

Hochheimer, M., and G. J. Unick. 2022. Systematic review and meta-analysis of retention in treatment using medications for opioid use disorder by medication, race/ethnicity, and gender in the United States. *Addictive Behaviors* 124:107113.

Hunter, S. B., A. R. Dopp, A. J. Ober, and L. Uscher-Pines. 2021. Clinician perspectives on methadone service delivery and the use of telemedicine during the COVID-19 pandemic: A qualitative study. *Journal of Substance Abuse Treatment* 124(May):108288. https://doi.org/10.1016/j.jsat.2021.108288.

Jones, C. M., M. Campopiano, G. Baldwin, and E. McCance-Katz. 2015. National and state treatment need and capacity for opioid agonist medication-assisted treatment. *American Journal of Public Health* 105(8):e55–e63. https://doi.org/10.2105/AJPH.2015.302664.

Joseph, G., K. Torres-Lockhart, M. R. Stein, P. A. Mund, and S. Nahvi. 2021. Reimagining patient-centered care in opioid treatment programs: Lessons from the Bronx during COVID-19. *Journal of Substance Abuse Treatment* 122(March):108219. https://doi.org/10.1016/j.jsat.2020.108219.

Joudrey, P. J., E. J. Edelman, and E. A. Wang. 2019a. Drive times to opioid treatment programs in urban and rural counties in 5 US states. *Journal of the American Medicine Association* 322(13):1310–1312. https://doi.org/10.1001/jama.2019.12562.

Joudrey, P. J., M. R. Khan, E. A. Wang, J. D. Scheidell, E. J. Edelman, D. K. McInnes, and A. D. Fox. 2019b. A conceptual model for understanding post-release opioid-related overdose risk. *Addiction Science & Clinical Practice* 14(1):17. https://doi.org/10.1186/s13722-019-0145-5.

Joudrey, P. J., N. Chadi, P. Roy, K. L. Morford, P. Bach, S. Kimmel, E. A. Wang, and S. L. Calcaterra. 2020. Pharmacy-based methadone dispensing and drive time to methadone treatment in five states within the United States: A cross-sectional study. *Drug and Alcohol Dependence* 211(March):107968. https://doi.org/10.1016/j.drugalcdep.2020.107968.

Kecojevic, A., C. F. Wong, S. M. Schrager, K. Silva, J. J. Bloom, E. Iverson, and S. E. Lankenau. 2012. Initiation into prescription drug misuse: Differences between lesbian, gay, bisexual, transgender (LGBT) and heterosexual high-risk young adults in Los Angeles and New York. *Addictive Behaviors* 37(11):1289–1293. https://doi.org/10.1016/j.addbeh.2012.06.006.

Kecojevic, A., C. F. Wong, H. L. Corliss, and S. E. Lankenau. 2015. Risk factors for high levels of prescription drug misuse and illicit drug use among substance-using young men who have sex with men (YMSM). *Drug and Alcohol Dependence* 150(May):156–163. https://doi.org/10.1016/j.drugalcdep.2015.02.031.

Keuroghlian, A. S. 2021. Electronic health records as an equity tool for LGBTQIA+ people. *Nature Medicine* 27(12):2071–2073. https://doi.org/10.1038/s41591-021-01592-3.

Keuroghlian, A. S., S. L. Reisner, J. M. White, and R. D. Weiss. 2015. Substance use and treatment of substance use disorders in a community sample of transgender adults. *Drug and Alcohol Dependence* 152:139–146.

Khatri, U. G., and T. N. A. Winkelman. 2022. Strengthening the Medicaid Reentry Act—supporting the health of people who are incarcerated. *The New England Journal of Medicine*, January. https://doi.org/10.1056/NEJMp2119571.

Kidorf, M., R. K. Brooner, K. E. Dunn, J. M. Peirce. 2021. Use of an electronic pillbox to increase number of methadone take-home doses during the COVID-19 pandemic. *Journal of Substance Abuse Treatment* 126:108328.

Kimmel, S. D., S. Rosenmoss, B. Bearnot, M. Larochelle, and A. Y. Walley. 2021. Rejection of patients with opioid use disorder referred for post-acute medical care before and after an anti-discrimination settlement in Massachusetts. *Journal of Addiction Medicine* 15(1):20–26. https://doi.org/10.1097/ADM.0000000000000693.

King, V. L., M. S. Kidorf, K. B. Stoller, R. Schwartz, K. Kolodner, and R. K. Brooner. 2006. A 12-month controlled trial of methadone medical maintenance integrated into an adaptive treatment model. *Journal of Substance Abuse Treatment* 31(4):385–393. https://doi.org/10.1016/j.jsat.2006.05.014.

Kleinman, R. A. 2020. Comparison of driving times to opioid treatment programs and pharmacies in the US. *Journal of American Medicine Association Psychiatry* 77(11):1163–1171. https://doi.org/10.1001/jamapsychiatry.2020.1624.

Krawczyk, N., H. Maniates, E. Hulsey, J. S. Smith, E. DiDomenico, E. A. Stuart, B. Saloner, and S. Bandara. 2022. Shifting medication treatment practices in the COVID-19 pandemic: A statewide survey of Pennsylvania opioid treatment programs. *Journal of Addiction Medicine*, February. https://doi.org/10.1097/ADM.0000000000000981.

Laks, J., J. Kehoe, N. M. Farrell, M. Komaromy, J. Kolodziej, A. Y. Walley, and J. L. Taylor. 2021. Methadone initiation in a bridge clinic for opioid withdrawal and opioid treatment program linkage: A case report applying the 72-hour rule. *Addiction Science & Clinical Practice* 16(1):73. https://doi.org/10.1186/s13722-021-00279-x.

Larochelle M. R., R. Bernstein, D. Bernson, T. Land, T. J. Stopka, A. J. Rose, M. Bharel, J. M. Liebschutz, and A. Y. Walley. 2019. Touchpoints—Opportunities to predict and prevent opioid overdose: A cohort study. *Drug and Alcohol Dependence* 1(204):107537. https://doi.org/10.1016/j.drugalcdep.2019.06.039.

Levander, X. A., J.D. Pytell, K. B. Stoller, P.T. Korthuis, G. Chander. 2021a. COVID-19-related policy changes for methadone take-home dosing: A multistate survey of opioid treatment program leadership. *Substance Abuse* 43(1):633–639.

Levander, X. A., K. A. Hoffman, J. W. McIlveen, D. McCarty, J. P. Terashima, and P. T. Korthuis. 2021b. Rural opioid treatment program patient perspectives on take-home methadone policy changes during COVID-19: A qualitative thematic analysis. *Addiction Science & Clinical Practice* 16(1):1–10.

Lintzeris, N., M. Lenne, and A. Ritter. 1999. Methadone injecting in Australia: A tale of two cities. *Addiction* 94(8):1175-1178.

Madden, E. F., B. T. Christian, P. A. Lagisetty, B. R. Ray, S. H. Sulzer. 2021. Treatment provider perceptions of take-home methadone regulation before and during COVID-19. *Drug and Alcohol Dependence* 228:109100.

Matheson, C. 1998. Privacy and stigma in the pharmacy: Illicit drug users' perspectives and implications for pharmacy practice. *Pharmaceutical Journal* 260(6992):639–641.

Matheson, C., C. M. Bond, and J. Pitcairn. 2002. Community pharmacy services for drug misusers in Scotland: What difference does 5 years make? *Addiction* 97(11):1405–1411. doi: 10.1046/j.1360-0443.2002.00241.x. PMID: 12410781.

McCarty, D., C. Bougatsos, B. Chan, K. A. Hoffman, K. C. Priest, S. Grusing, and R. Chou. 2021. Office-based methadone treatment for opioid use disorder and pharmacy dispensing: A scoping review. *The American Journal of Psychiatry* 178(9):804–817. https://doi.org/10.1176/appi.ajp.2021.20101548.

Minton, T. D., L. G. Beatty, and Z. Zeng. 2021. Correctional populations in the United States, 2019—Statistical Tables. U.S. Department of Justice, Office of Justice Programs, Bureau of Justice Statistics: NCJ:300655. https://bjs.ojp.gov/sites/g/files/xyckuh236/files/media/document/cpus19st.pdf (accessed May 9, 2022).

NASEM (National Academies of Sciences, Engineering, and Medicine). 2019. *Medications for opioid use disorder save lives*. Washington, DC: The National Academies Press.

Neale, J. 1999. Drug users' views of substitute prescribing conditions. *International Journal of Drug Policy* 10(3):247-258. https://doi.org/10.1097/01.adt.0000210713.80198.d1.

Neale, J., C. N. E. Tompkins, R. McDonald, and J. Strang. 2018. Patient views of opioid pharmacotherapy biodelivery systems: Qualitative study to assist treatment decision making. *Experimental and Clinical Psychopharmacology* 26(6):570–581. https://doi.org/10.1037/pha0000217.

NIDA (National Institute on Drug Abuse). 2021. Medications to treat opioid disorder research report: How much does opioid treatment cost? https://nida.nih.gov/publications/research-reports/medications-to-treat-opioid-addiction/how-much-does-opioid-treatment-cost (accessed June 12, 2022).

Nielsen, S., A. Cheetham, J, Jackson, S. Lord, D. Petrie, D. Jacka, L. Picco, and K. Morgan. 2021. A prospective, multisite implementation-efficacy trial of a collaborative prescriber-pharmacist model of care for medication assisted treatment for opioid dependence: Protocol for the EPIC-MATOD study. *Research in Social and Administration Pharmarcy* S1551-7411(21)00379-X. https://doi.org/10.1016/j.sapharm.2021.11.007. Epub ahead of print. PMID: 34924314

Peavy, K. M., J. Darnton, P. Grekin, M. Russo, C. J. B. Green, J. O. Merrill, C. Fontinos, S. Woolworth, S. Soth, J. I. Tsui. 2020. Rapid implementation of service delivery changes to mitigate COVID-19 and maintain access to methadone among persons with and at high-risk for HIV in an opioid treatment program. *AIDS and Behavior* 24(9):2469–2472.

Qato, D. M., S. Zenk, J. Wilder, R. Harrington, D. Gaskin, G. C. Alexander. 2017. The availability of pharmacies in the United States: 2007–2015. *PloS One* 12:e0183172.

Ranapurwala, S. I., M. E. Shanahan, A. A. Alexandridis, S. K. Proescholdbell, R. B. Naumann, D. Edwards, S. W. Marshall. 2018. Opioid overdose mortality among former North Carolina inmates: 2000–2015. *American Journal of Public Health* 108(9):1207–1213.

Rieckmann, T., L. Moore, C. Croy, G. A. Aarons, and D. K. Novins. 2017. National overview of medication-assisted treatment for American Indians and Alaska Natives with substance use disorders. *Psychiatric Services* (Washington, DC) 68(11):1136–1143. https://doi.org/10.1176/appi.ps.201600397.

SAMHSA (Substance Abuse and Mental Health Services Administration). 2015. Federal guidelines for opioid treatment programs. https://store.samhsa.gov/product/Federal-Guidelines-for-Opioid-Treatment-Programs/PEP15-FEDGUIDEOTP (accessed April 26, 2022).

SAMHSA. 2019. Key substance use and mental health indications in the United States: Results from the 2018 National Survey on Drug Use and Health. (HHS Publication No. PEP19-5068, NSDUH Series H-54). https://www.samhsa.gov/data (accessed April 26, 2022).

SAMHSA. 2020. Medications for opioid use disorder: Treatment protocol (Tip) Series 63. https://store.samhsa.gov/sites/default/files/SAMHSA_Digital_Download/PEP20-02-01-006.pdf (accessed May 6, 2022).

SAMHSA. 2021. Key substance use and mental health indicators in the United States: Results from the 2020 National Survey on Drug Use and Health (HHS Publication No. PEP21-07-01-003, NSDUH Series H-56). Rockville, MD: Center for Behavioral Health Statistics and Quality, Substance Abuse and Mental Health Services Administration. Retrieved from https://www.samhsa.gov/data/ (accesed June 8, 2022).

Schiff, D. M., T. Nielsen, B. B. Hoeppner, M. Terplan, H. Hansen, D. Bernson, H. Diop, M. Bharel, E. E. Krans, S. Selk, J. F. Kelly, T. E. Wilens, and E. M. Taveras. 2020. Assessment of racial and ethnic disparities in the use of medication to treat opioid use disorder among pregnant women in Massachusetts. *Journal of American Medicine Association* 3(5)e205734. https://doi.org/10.1001/jamanetworkopen.2020.5734.

Scott, C.K., M. L. Dennis, C. E. Grella, A. F. Mischel, and J. Carnevale. 2021. The impact of the opioid crisis on U.S. state prison systems. *Health Justice* 9:17. https://doi.org/10.1186/s40352-021-00143-9Senay, E. C., A. G. Barthwell, R. Marks, P. Bokos, D. Gillman, R. White, and C. A. Pristach. 1993. Medical maintenance: A pilot study. *Journal of Addictive Diseases* 12(4):59–76.

Strang, J., W. Hall, M. Hickman, and S. M. Bird. 2010. Impact of supervision of methadone consumption on deaths related to methadone overdose (1993-2008): Analyses using OD4 index in England and Scotland. *British Medical Journal* 341:c4851 doi:10.1136/bmj.c485 - https://www.bmj.com/content/341/bmj.c4851Suen, L. W., S. Castellanos, N. Joshi, S. Satterwhite, and K. R. Knight. 2021. "The idea is to help people achieve greater success and liberty": A qualitative study of expanded methadone take-home access in opioid use disorder treatment. *medRxiv*. https://doi.org/10.1101/2021.08.20.21262382.

Taylor, J. L., J. Laks, P. J. Christine, J. Kehoe, J. Evans, T. W. Kim, N. M. Farrell, C. S. White, Z. M. Weinstein, and A. Y. Walley. 2022. Bridge clinic implementation of "72-hour rule" methadone for opioid withdrawal management: Impact on opioid treatment program linkage and retention in care. *Drug and Alcohol Dependence* 236:109497.

Tran A. D., R. Chen, S. Nielsen, E. Zahra, L. Degenhardt, T. Santo, M. Farrell, and B. Larance. 2022. Economic analysis of out-of-pocket costs among people in opioid agonist treatment: A cross-sectional survey in three Australian jurisdictions. *International Journal of Drug Policy* 99:103472. doi: 10.1016/j.drugpo.2021.103472.

Trowbridge, P., Z. M. Weinstein, T. Kerensky, P. Roy, D. Regan, J. H. Samet, and A. Y. Walley. 2017. Addiction consultation services—Linking hospitalized patients to outpatient addiction treatment. *Journal of Substance Abuse Treatment* 79(August):1–5. https://doi.org/10.1016/j.jsat.2017.05.007.

U.S. Census Bureau. 2012. 2010 Census show nearly half of American Indians and Alaska Natives report multiple races. Newsroom Archive. https://www.census.gov/newsroom/releases/archives/2010_census/cb12-cn06.html (accesed June 12, 2022).

Wagner, P., and B. Rabuy. 2017. Following the money of mass incarceration. *Prison Policy Initiative*, January 25. https://www.prisonpolicy.org/reports/money.html (accessed June 12, 2022).

Walley, A. Y., S. Lodi, Y. Li, D. Bernson, H. Babakhanlou-Chase, T. Land, and M. R. Larochelle. 2020. Association between mortality rates and medication and residential treatment after in-patient medically managed opioid withdrawal: A cohort analysis. *Addiction (Abingdon, England)* 115(8):1496–1508. https://doi.org/10.1111/add.14964.

White, W. L., C. K. Scott, M. L. Dennis, and M. G. Boyle. 2005. It's time to stop kicking people out of addiction treatment. *Counselor* (Deerfield Beach, FL) 6(2):12.

Winkelman, T. N. A., V. W. Chang, and I. A. Binswanger. 2018. Health, polysubstance use, and criminal justice involvement among adults with varying levels of opioid use. *Journal of American Medicine Association* 1(3):e180558. https://doi.org/10.1001/jamanetworkopen.2018.0558.

Wu, L., H. Zhu, and M. S. Swartz. 2016. Treatment utilization among persons with opioid use disorder in the United States. *Drug and Alcohol Dependence* 169(December):117–127. https://doi.org/10.1016/j.drugalcdep.2016.10.015.

Wu, L., W. S. John, U. E. Ghitza, A. Wahle, A. G. Matthews, M. Lewis, B. Hart, Z. Hubbard, L. A. Bowlby, L. H. Greenblatt, and P. Mannelli. 2021. Buprenorphine physician–pharmacist collaboration in the management of patients with opioid use disorder: Results from a multisite study of the National Drug Abuse Treatment Clinical Trials Network. *Addiction (Abingdon, England)* 116(7):1805–1816. https://doi.org/10.1111/add.15353.

Wu, L., W. S. John, E. D. Morse, S. Adkins, J. Pippin, R. K. Brooner, and R. P. Schwartz. 2022. Opioid treatment program and community pharmacy collaboration for methadone maintenance treatment: Results from a feasibility clinical trial. *Addiction* 117(2):444–456. https://doi.org/10.1111/add.15641.

Zeng, Z. 2020. Jail inmates in 2018. U.S. Department of Justice, Office of Justice Programs, Bureau of Justice Statistics. https://bjs.ojp.gov/library/publications/jail-inmates-2018 (accessed May 9, 2022).

Zule, W. A., C. Oramasionwu, D. Evon, S. Hino, I. A. Doherty, G. V. Bobashev, and W. M. Wechsberg. 2016. Event-level analyses of sex-risk and injection-risk behaviors among nonmedical prescription opioid users. *The American Journal of Drug and Alcohol Abuse* 42(6):689–697. https://doi.org/10.1080/00952990.2016.1174706.

B

Workshop Agenda

Methadone Treatment for Opioid Use Disorder:
Examining Federal Regulations and Laws
A Workshop

March 3–4, 2022 | Virtual

Workshop Objectives:

A planning committee of the National Academies of Sciences, Engineering, and Medicine will organize and conduct a 2-day public workshop that brings together experts and key stakeholders to examine the current federal regulatory and legal landscape regarding provision of and access to methadone for the treatment of opioid use disorder.

Invited presentations and discussions will be designed to:

- Examine current federal regulations governing methadone treatment services, including the current COVID-19 emergency regulatory relief;
- Discuss the impact of these regulations relative to other factors affecting treatment services;
- Explore potential options for modifying federal regulations and laws to expand access to quality treatment with methadone; and
- Explore state laws that may conflict with federal regulations.

DAY 1: THURSDAY, MARCH 3, 2022

9:30am ET   **Welcome and Opening Remarks**
Alan Leshner, CEO Emeritus, American Association for the Advancement of Science; *Workshop Chair*

9:35am   **Opening Talks Highlighting Lived Experiences**
Abby Coulter, Urban Survivors Union; co-author of the *Methadone Manifesto*; *Planning Committee Member*
Walter Ginter, Medication Assisted Recovery Support Team
Brenda Davis, National Alliance for Medication Assisted Recovery, Inc.

SESSION 1: METHADONE TREATMENT AND REGULATION – HISTORICAL PERSPECTIVE AND OVERVIEW OF WHERE WE ARE TODAY

Session Objective: Examine the history and current status of methadone treatment and regulations in the United States.

Key Discussion Questions:
- How have methadone regulations evolved to where they are today?
- What are the effects of methadone regulation on health inequities, including social barriers to treatment, and the considerations for special populations?
- What are some of the federal priorities and collaborative efforts aimed at addressing longstanding barriers and improving access to quality treatment?

10:05am   **Session Overview**
Helena Hansen, University of California, Los Angeles; *Planning Committee Member; Session Moderator*

10:10am   **The Politics of Stigma and Racialization in the Early Years of Methadone Maintenance Regulation**
Samuel Kelton Roberts, Jr., Columbia University

10:25am   **Racial Disparities in Access, Initiation, and Retention in Methadone Treatment and Implications for Policy Formulation**
Magdalena Cerdá, New York University; *Planning Committee Member*

10:40am	Considerations for Special Populations and Circumstances
	• Pregnant/Parenting People
	    Mishka Terplan, Friends Research Institute
	
	• People Living with HIV & LGBTQIA+ Populations
	    Alex Keuroghlian, The Fenway Institute; Harvard Medical School
	
	• Older Adults
	    Ximena Levander, Oregon Health & Science University

11:10am	Moderated Discussion with the Speakers and Q&A
11:30am	**BREAK**
11:40am	ONDCP Presentation – Goals and Priorities of the Administration Rahul Gupta, Director, Office of National Drug Control Policy, Executive Office of the President

11:50am	Overview of the Current Regulatory Landscape and Flexible Responses during COVID-19
	• U.S. Department of Health and Human Services (HHS)
	    Rebecca Haffajee, Acting Assistant Secretary for Planning and Evaluation
	
	• Substance Abuse and Mental Health Services Administration (SAMHSA)
	    Yngvild Olsen, Acting Director of the Center for Substance Abuse Treatment
	
	• Drug Enforcement Administration (DEA)
	    Kristi O'Malley, Special Advisor to the Administrator

12:20am	Lessons Learned from COVID-19 and Regulatory Change in the Wake of Necessity Noa Krawczyk, New York University

12:35pm	Overview of The Pew Charitable Trusts' 50-State Analysis of Methadone Regulations **Frances McGaffey,** The Pew Charitable Trusts
12:45pm	Moderated Discussion with the Speakers and Q&A
1:05pm	**LUNCH**

SESSION 2: IMPROVING ACCESS TO QUALITY TREATMENT IN OTPS THROUGH REGULATORY INNOVATION

Session Objective: Explore broad implementation of innovations, supported by evidence, and best practices to ensure access and quality treatment in opioid treatment programs (OTPs): What is allowed now and what requires regulatory change?

Key Discussion Questions:
- What innovations and best practices, including those from the COVID-19 pandemic, could be more broadly implemented within the existing regulatory framework to support a) access, b) quality, and c) safety?
  - What evidence is available regarding the effect of regulatory innovation and flexibility implemented during the COVID-19 pandemic?
  - Other opportunities for regulatory flexibility
- What potentially useful innovations would require formal rulemaking or legislative action?
  - What specifically would that look like?
- What steps would enhance health equity?

1:40pm	Session Overview **Ken Stoller,** Johns Hopkins University; *Planning Committee Member; Session Moderator*
1:45pm	Legal Analysis **Bridget Dooling,** George Washington University; *Planning Committee Member*
2:00pm	Pharmacy Dispensing as an Extension of OTPs **Robert Brooner,** Friends Research Institute
2:15pm	Mobile Units **Valerie Mielke,** New Jersey Department of Human Services

APPENDIX B

2:30pm OTPs as Hub Sites in Systemic Expansion
         Mark Parrino, American Association for the Treatment of
             Opioid Dependence, Inc.

2:45pm Moderated Discussion with the Speakers and Q&A

3:10pm BREAK

SESSION 3: IMPROVING ACCESS TO QUALITY TREATMENT IN THE CRIMINAL JUSTICE SYSTEM AND OTHER INSTITUTIONAL SETTINGS

Session Objective: Explore possible regulatory initiatives at the federal level that would improve access to quality treatment with methadone in federal, state, and local correctional settings, and in other institutional settings.

Key Discussion Questions:
- What available discretion in existing regulations could be better leveraged to support a) access, b) quality, and c) safety in institutional settings?
- What evidence is available regarding the effect of the innovations and regulatory flexibility implemented during the COVID-19 pandemic?
- What regulatory (or statutory?) changes at the federal level are needed to improve access and quality in federal, state, and local institutional settings? What exactly would that look like?
- What steps would enhance health equity?

3:25pm Session Overview
         Tracie Gardner, Legal Action Center, *Planning Committee
             Member; Session Moderator*

3:30pm **Crosscutting Regulatory Issues that Impact Corrections Facilities at All Levels and Other Institutions**
         Josiah "Jody" Rich, Brown University; *Planning Committee
             Member*

3:45pm **Transitional Clinic Networks**
         Emily Wang, Yale School of Medicine

4:00pm	A State Trial Court Perspective Judge Michael Barrasse, Lackawanna County Court of Common Pleas, Pennsylvania
4:15pm	Civil Rights Litigation to Enable Methadone Treatment in Institutions Rachael Rollins and Greg Dorchak, U.S. States Attorneys' Offices–Massachusetts
4:30pm	Moderated Discussion with the Speakers and Q&A
4:55pm	Day 1 Closing Remarks Alan Leshner, CEO Emeritus, American Association for the Advancement of Science; *Workshop Chair*
5:00pm	ADJOURN

DAY 2: Friday, March 4, 2022

9:30am	Welcome and Recap of Day 1 Alan Leshner, CEO Emeritus, American Association for the Advancement of Science; *Workshop Chair*

SESSION 4: EXPANDING ACCESS TO METHADONE THROUGH REGULATORY INNOVATION

Session Objective: Explore broad implementation of innovations, supported by evidence, and best practices to ensure access and quality treatment using models and settings other than OTPs: What is allowed now and what requires regulatory change?

Key Discussion Questions:
- What innovations and best practices involving models and settings other than OTPs could be implemented more broadly within the existing regulatory framework to support a) access, b) quality, and c) safety?
    - Are there available regulatory opportunities not currently understood or leveraged?
- What innovations require formal rulemaking or legislative action?
    - What concretely would that look like?
- What steps would enhance health equity?

9:40am	Session Overview **Gavin Bart,** Hennepin Healthcare; University of Minnesota Medical School; *Planning Committee Member; Session Moderator*
9:45am	**Office-Based Methadone** **Robert Schwartz,** Friends Research Institute
10:00am	**Pharmacy-Based Dispensing** **Li-Tzy Wu,** Duke University School of Medicine
10:15am	**International Models of Pharmacy-Based Dispensing** **Janie Sheridan,** University of Auckland **Suzanne Nielsen,** Monash University
10:30am	**Innovative Models of Initiation under Existing Regulations – Inpatient and Outpatient Settings** **Alexander Walley,** Boston University and Massachusetts Department of Public Health
10:45am	**Potential New Treatment Modalities/Settings that Could be Opened up with Regulatory Changes** **Ayana Jordan,** New York University **Kamilla Venner,** University of New Mexico
11:15am	**BREAK**
11:30am	**Regulatory Opportunities to Remove Current Barriers** **Corey Davis,** The Network for Public Health Law
11:45am	**Regulatory Incentives to Facilitate Access to Quality Treatment** **Matthew Lawrence,** Emory University School of Law; *Planning Committee Member*
12:00pm	Moderated Discussion with the Speakers and Q&A
12:45pm	**LUNCH**

SESSION 5: ASSESSING POTENTIAL LEGAL AND REGULATORY CHANGES

Session Objective: Explore a framework that might guide the assessment of potential legal and regulatory changes that would yield the most benefit for improving access to quality methadone treatment for all.

Key Discussion Question:
- How can the potential impact of the different regulatory mechanisms discussed throughout the workshop be assessed and prioritized? For example:
  o When considering the evidence, how many more people might have access to treatment?
  o What might the health outcomes be, and at what cost?
  o What inroads can such actions make on health equity?
  o How can a framework address both public health and diversion concerns?

1:30pm	Overview **Alan Leshner,** CEO Emeritus, American Association for the Advancement of Science; *Workshop Chair; Session Moderator*
1:35pm	A Policy Analysis Framework to Support Health Policy Decisions **Richard Frank,** Harvard Medical School; The Brookings Institution
1:55pm	A Cost-Effectiveness Framework to Assess Potential Legal and Regulatory Changes **Michael French,** University of Miami
2:15pm	Moderated Discussion with Speakers and Q&A
2:35pm	**BREAK**
2:50pm	Synthesis and Prioritization of Legal and Regulatory Actions **Richard Bonnie,** University of Virginia, *Planning Committee Member*

APPENDIX B   *133*

3:00pm   **Panel Discussion on Concrete Actions**
            John Brooklyn, BAART St. Albans and Howard Center
                Burlington Vermont
            Chinazo Cunningham, New York State Office of Addiction
                Services and Supports
            David Frank, New York University
            Joy Rucker, Former Executive Director, Texas Harm
                Reduction Alliance
            Brendan Saloner, Johns Hopkins University
            Shelly Weizman, O'Neill Institute for National and Global
                Health Law, Georgetown Law

3:45pm   **Audience Q&A**

4:25pm   **Acknowledgments and Concluding Remarks**
            Alan Leshner, CEO Emeritus, American Association for the
                Advancement of Science; *Workshop Chair*

4:30pm   **ADJOURN WORKSHOP**

Appendix C

Commissioned Papers

The Politics of Stigma and Racialization in the Early Years of Methadone Maintenance Regulation

Samuel Kelton Roberts, PhD*
Associate Professor of History & Sociomedical Sciences
Columbia University
322 Fayerweather Hall, MC2519
1180 Amsterdam Avenue
skroberts@columbia.edu

INTRODUCTION

Social science researchers have established structural racism and stigma against methadone maintenance patients as a barrier to recruitment and retention of people of color in need of treatment. Structural racism — enacted through a broad array of institutional practices and policy decisions — negatively impacts effective treatment by influencing the terms on which Black patients might gain access and successfully engage in the therapeutic process. Stigma has the deleterious effect of alienating patients and potential patients from a valuable source of help — Black patients, as Andraka-Christou has noted, suffer a "trifecta of stigmas" by virtue of being Black, having an opioid use disorder, and being a methadone patient.[1] Researchers who focus on structural barriers to access and popular stigma against methadone maintenance treatment (MMT) make the argument that in no case are matters made better by the onerous restrictions on methadone and the regimes of surveillance required by federal regulation. Even today, methadone maintenance remains one of the nation's most closely regulated medical protocols. Perhaps not entirely by coincidence, it is also one of the most stigmatized, controversial, and misunderstood.[2]

---

* The author is responsible for the content of this article, which does not necessarily represent the views of the National Academies of Sciences, Engineering, and Medicine.

[1] Barbara Andraka-Christou, "Addressing Racial and Ethnic Disparities in the Use of Medications for Opioid Use Disorder," *Health Affairs* 40, no. 6 (2021).

[2] Bennett Allen, Michelle L. Nolan, and Denise Paone, "Underutilization of Medications to Treat Opioid Use Disorder: What Role Does Stigma Play?," *Substance Abuse* 40, no. 4 (2019); Holly N. Hagle et al., "Dismantling Racism against Black, Indigenous, and People of Color across the Substance Use Continuum: A Position Statement of the Association for Multidisciplinary Education and Research in Substance Use and Addiction," *Substance abuse* 42, no. 1 (2021); Anastasia Hudgins et al., "Barriers to Effective Care: Specialty Drug Treatment in Philadelphia," *Journal of substance abuse treatment* 131 (2021); Kelly Ray Knight, *Addicted.Pregnant.Poor* (Durham, NC: Duke University Press, 2015); Brendan Saloner et al., "A Public Health Strategy for the Opioid Crisis," *Public health reports (1974)* 133, no. 1S (2018); Alexander C. Tsai et al., "Stigma as a Fundamental Hindrance to the United States Opioid Overdose Crisis Response," *PLoS medicine* 16, no. 11 (2019); Tricia H. Witte et al., "Stigma Surrounding the Use of Medically Assisted Treatment for Opioid Use Disorder," *Substance Use & Misuse* 56, no. 10 (2021); Lindsay Wolfson et al., "Examining Barriers to Harm Reduction and Child Welfare Services for Pregnant Women and Mothers Who Use Substances Using a Stigma Action Framework," *Health & social care in the*

APPENDIX C

    In this paper, I specifically examine the historical origins of methadone stigma in the context of Black American *political culture*. In doing so, I argue that Black Americans' antimethadone attitudes, first formed in the late 1960s, emerged from methadone's political history in this country and, also, the much longer history of medical disrespect and abuse of Black Americans. For Black and White liberals in the 1960s and 1970s, issues of major concern included community control of local institutions such as school boards, medical clinics, and antipoverty programs; civil and economic rights for all Americans; youth alienation; policing reform; and the war in Vietnam. More importantly, they tended to view all of these as being closely linked and in some way causally related to another concern: the growing problem of heroin addiction among Black and Latino Americans. From this point of view, methadone maintenance appeared to address only an individual's dependence on heroin, not the broader social conditions that produced drug addiction among large groups of people. Distrust seemed warranted for another reason as well. In less than two decades, Americans had witnessed astounding revelations of government complicity in a wide range of medical abuses, including coerced sterilization of Black, Latina, and Native women of color; harassment and infiltration of prominent civil rights organizations; and, in the early 1970s, the Tuskegee syphilis study on rural, poor Black men and their sexual partners, and medical experimentation on incarcerated men in Holmesburg Prison in Pennsylvania. The capacity for abuse by a system designed to keep heavily surveilled patients indefinitely dependent on a narcotic supplied by clinics that were largely outside of community control was not simply potential, but actual. In many municipalities there were poor Black and White patients who reported having joined programs as a requirement of parole or probation or in exchange for welfare benefits.

    In this light, popular distrust of MMT was lamentable, but entirely understandable. However, that distrust was in some ways misplaced, as it was *methadone policy and politics*, not anything inherent to the drug itself, which were most problematic. I focus mainly on how the era's politics helped to produce federal regulatory policy in the early 1970s, which inadvertently served to make methadone maintenance much more polarizing that it had to be. Those policies remained in place until the mid-1990s, with many aspects still existing today. The unfortunate result is that, 50 years after the first Food and Drug Administration (FDA) MMT regulations, structural barriers and popular stigma against methadone maintenance and its patients are powerful deterrents to those seeking help.

    I begin by briefly outlining the early years of methadone maintenance politics and policy, from roughly 1969 to 1975, to show how the FDA responded to multiple concerns regarding addiction and drug-related crime, methadone's actual ability to rehabilitate, the possibility of street diversion, and the potential for government abuse and social control. At greater length I elaborate on the points of contention specifically from Black and White critics whose opposition was philosophical and political. I conclude with a discussion about the paths not taken during this period.

---

community 29, no. 3 (2021); Julia Woo et al., "'Don't Judge a Book by Its Cover': A Qualitative Study of Methadone Patients' Experiences of Stigma," *Substance Abuse: Research and Treatment* 11 (2017); Kyaien O. Conner et al., "It's Like Night and Day. He's White. I'm Black: Shared Stigmas between Counselors and Older Adult Methadone Clients," *Best Practices in Mental Health* 6, no. 1 (2010); Kyaien O. Conner and Daniel Rosen, "'You're Nothing but a Junkie': Multiple Experiences of Stigma in an Aging Methadone Maintenance Population," *Journal of Social Work Practice in the Addictions* 8, no. 2 (2008).

The Regulatory Mire

I have noted elsewhere methadone maintenance's convoluted regulatory history. It was in mid-1970 when MM first entered FDA regulatory purview, only weeks after the Nixon administration communicated its own support for MMT expansion. Federal guidelines before this had permitted the use of methadone only in analgesia and medically supervised withdrawal of opioid-addicted patients. Addressing the emergence of maintenance, novel guidelines promulgated by the FDA and the Federal Bureau of Narcotics and Dangerous Drugs (BNDD conferred on methadone investigational new drug (IND) status for maintenance purposes, in which practitioners were bound by requirements in licensing; maximum daily dosage; diversion prevention; strict recordkeeping; staff supervision; applicant screening; patient monitoring for abuse of other drugs (urine testing); and provision of ancillary services (e.g., counseling, psychotherapy, and vocational assistance). Excluded from treatment were minors, pregnant women, and persons suffering from psychosis or from extreme physical disability.[3]

Many hailed the new regulation as a major advance in addiction treatment as it would, so it was presumed, standardize treatment across the country. Yet some physicians believed the regulations tied their hands. Several had opened clinics that had thrived during the recent years of ambiguous regulation. Those who did not comply with the new regulations quickly found themselves under intense federal scrutiny.[4] Meanwhile, Dr. Vincent Dole, who with Dr. Marie Nyswander in New York brought methadone maintenance into being, was deeply bothered that the FDA and BNDD had constructed the June 1970 model protocol "with essentially no consultation with knowledgeable people in the field." Even the provisions that most of the public would have thought reasonable were, in Dole's opinion, countertherapeutic. In excluding from the model protocol patients deemed psychotic, the FDA had deprived physicians of the opportunity to treat an otherwise unreachable population and to add other psychiatric treatments to methadone. He offered a similar argument regarding those with physical illness, arguing that, for example, before methadone maintenance, hard-core heroin users with tuberculosis "would be running off all the time without taking their medicine for tuberculosis." In the context of a methadone clinic, however, such patients could be issued both. Even the concern regarding the effects of methadone on pregnancy missed the point. Dole asserted that he had treated many women whose pregnancies were entirely normal while on methadone, but worried that these women otherwise would have continued to use heroin had they been denied the treatment.[5]

Less than a year later, in early April 1971, the FDA relaxed its regulations on methadone maintenance, upgrading its status from an "investigative new drug" to a "new drug application." Gone were those provisions of the 1970 model protocol, which excluded pregnant women, people under the age of 18 years, and those with physical or mental illness. Additionally, private physicians also were allowed to dispense methadone on a maintenance basis. Of equal importance, politically as well as therapeutically, clinics no longer had to limit daily dose to 160 milligrams. Nor were they required to stipulate for each patient an eventual goal of narcotic addiction "cure," the complete independence from any opioid at all, including methadone. With the lowering of exclusions and the elongation of treatment duration to a perhaps indefinite period

---

[3] Helena Hansen and Samuel Roberts, "Two Tiers of Biomedicalization: Buprenorphine, Methadone and the Biopolitics of Addiction Stigma and Race," in *Critical Perspectives on Addiction*, ed. Julie Netherland (Bingley, UK: Emerald, 2012).

[4] David Courtwright, Herman Joseph, and Don Des Jarlais, *Addicts Who Survived: An Oral History of Narcotic Use in America, 1923-1965* (Knoxville: University of Tennessee Press, 1989).

[5] "Methadone Plans Called Unworkable," *The Austin Statesman*, 13 July 1970.

of time, both the number of patients recruited and those retained ballooned. Funded largely by President Nixon's Special Action Office on Drug Abuse Prevention, the number of methadone maintenance patients in the United States grew from 9,100 to 73,000 between 1971 and 1973. Some estimates stated a figure as high as 85,000.

The lowered restrictions and the dramatic expansion of the patient ranks unnerved many. Lawmakers at every level of government expressed concern about reports of loose protocols, failure to offer other kinds of therapy in conjunction with methadone, inconsistent urine testing of patients, and street diversion of methadone. Many physicians found themselves the target of popular and official allegations of medical profiteering and even intentional street diversion. Some undoubtedly were. If newspaper accounts are to be believed, before 1972 (the years of office-based prescription), in any American city with physicians prescribing methadone, there might have been as many as two or more physicians under some kind of formal or informal investigation by the Bureau of Narcotics and Danger Drugs, the FDA, local law enforcement, or even health officials. Most either complied with authorities or quietly closed shop. Others, in cases which often rose to the level of national attention, defended themselves against charges in the courts of law or public opinion. Dr. Thomas Moore, an African-American physician practicing in Washington, DC, denied all charges of prolific prescribing and retorted that the rising demand for street heroin was a demonstration of the need for more availability of methadone. Other physicians made similar arguments. At hearings held in late 1972 and early 1973 by the Senate Subcommittee to Investigate Juvenile Delinquency, Roger Smith, the director of a multimodality addiction treatment program in San Rafael (Marin County), CA, testified that he was not that concerned about diversion and suggested that measures to curb it could do more harm than good in that they would work against patient recruitment and retention. San Rafael is not far from San Francisco, whose Sheriff, Richard Hongisto, also questioned the assumption that diversion represented a social threat while expressing the opinion that the British system of heroin maintenance and the U.S. system of methadone maintenance were "a more humane and cheaper response than continual criminalization."[6]

Some of the April 1971 relaxations were retracted a year later, in early April 1972, when the FDA again decided that children below age 18 should not be treated with methadone. In the 1972 regulations, the FDA also restricted methadone prescription to "a closed system" of clinics in which new patients in their first 3 months would be closely supervised when administered methadone. Physicians no longer could prescribe methadone from their office for a patient to purchase at a local pharmacy, and patients, even after their 3-month probationary period, would not be allowed to take home more than a 3-day supply. To further ensure patient compliance, the FDA mandated weekly urinalysis tests to monitor polydrug use. At the same time, however, the FDA imposed a hybrid set of guidelines (combining both IND and NDA status) and approved methadone for narcotic addiction treatment, a move that further expanded the ranks of patients. These new guidelines became effective 90 days later, only to be altered again under the Narcotic Addict Treatment Act of 1974, which gave increased regulatory and investigative authority to the BNDD's successor, the Drug Enforcement Administration (DEA).[7]

---

[6] *Methadone Use and Abuse -- 1972-73. Hearings before the Subcommittee to Investigate Juvenile Delinquency of the Senate Committee on the Judiciary; November 14 and 16, 1972; February 8, 13, and 14, and April 6, 1973*, Second Session of the 92nd Congress and First Session of the 93rd Congress, 1973, 271-72.

[7] Ida Walters, "Curse or Cure?," *Wall Street Journal*, 27 July 1972; Henry L. Lennard, Leon J. Epstein, and Mitchell S. Rosenthal, "The Methadone Illusion," *Science* 176, no. 4037 (1972). On the history of FDA regulation, see Philip J. Hilts, *Protecting America's Health: The Fda, Business, and One Hundred Years of Regulation* (New York: Alfred A. Knopf, 2003).

The Making of a Controversy

In announcing its guidelines, nothing in the FDA's language forecasted its role in the major racial controversy it helped to create. There were, of course, no provisos regarding ethnic composition of the patient base or the clinical personnel. However, in their extreme vigilance to prevent street diversion, to mandate urine testing to discourage patient "cheating" (using other drugs while on methadone), and to regulate physician practice and surveil patients, the FDA and BNDD produced a regulatory environment in which the treatment protocol was limited only to a specialized set of mainly White physicians, effectively alienating Black communities and even Black physicians. In a matter of just a few years, a fairly dominant consensus in the Black public sphere viewed methadone maintenance as anathema to the main political programs of the previous two decades.

Although in Black political culture methadone maintenance has held a generally unenviable place of distrust and derision, Black opinion on methadone or narcotic maintenance was not monolithically negative, nor was it uniformly consistent over time. As early as 1953, in answer to the question, "Should Dope Be Legalized?," the editors of the Black middle-class *Ebony* magazine gave serious consideration to proposals for private and government-run heroin and morphine maintenance clinics.[8] In 1963, the grassroots Harlem Neighborhoods Association, Inc. (HANA) declared that it "views addiction as a *medical problem*" not to be "viewed as a moral defect, and an occasion for great shame." It also pointed to "the British system of legal availability of drugs to addicts," and called for reasoned consideration of "a limited program for the legalization of drugs," especially for those waiting to be admitted to rehabilitation programs.[9] In response to a 1964 New York City Council resolution to explore the possibility of narcotic maintenance (methadone was not specified), Rev. Eugene Callender, a prominent Harlem clergyperson and community organizer with a history of addiction outreach, sounded much like a proto-harm reductionist. The plan, which Callender called an "excellent idea" that should be tried in a 3-year pilot program, reminded him of the British system of narcotics maintenance. "At least," he said, "he [the addicted individual] would be getting good drugs, instead of the garbage he gets in the streets and which is given to him through dirty instruments."[10] Upon hearing the news of the Dole–Nyswander experiment in 1965, women's and civil rights activist Dorothy Height was cautiously optimistic: "Research on methadone is still in a very early stage, but it may lead to a new understanding and treatment of drug addicts. So far methadone has enabled some addicts, for the first time in their lives, to become self-supporting, responsible members of the community."[11] What changed between 1953 and the early 1970s was the political configurations surrounding narcotics maintenance, not the idea of narcotics maintenance itself.

The 1972 regulations had been designed to strike a balance of proponents and opponents of methadone maintenance who themselves represented a broad range of public concerns. The most ardent of supporters, often physicians, saw in methadone maintenance real rehabilitative

---

[8] "Should Dope Be Legalized? Doctors, Police and Social Workers Debate Drastic Move to Set up Legal Clinics as Step to Combat Narcotics Racket," *Ebony*, April 1953.

[9] Joseph P. King, Lonnie MacDonald, and Harlem Neighborhoods Association Inc. (HANA), "A Preliminary Report of the Neighborhood Conference on Narcotics Addiction, Co-Sponsored by Harlem Neighborhoods Association Mental Health Committee, Harlem Hospital Department of Psychiatry," (Malcolm X Papers, Schomburg Center for Black History and Culture; Box 10, Folder 14, 1963).

[10] "Clergymen Back, Hit Giving Dope to Addicts," *New York Amsterdam News* 22 February 1964.

[11] Dorothy Height, "A Woman's Word," *New York Amsterdam News*, 4 September 1965.

potential, especially when combined with counseling, social services, and vocational or educational assistance (historically, this combination of medically assisted treatment with supportive services has produced the best results). Allied with this group were those whose support for MMT emanated from concerns about escalating crime rates attributable, so they believed, to drug users. Meanwhile, methadone's critics were more diverse, united mainly in their opposition. For example, there were NIMBYist elements who worried mainly about declining property values and public safety in their neighborhoods. Similarly, by 1970 the "drug-free" (non-methadone) addiction rehabilitation industry was reaching its maturity, but few organizations in the field were so established as to not regard methadone maintenance as an ideologically and even economically competing threat.

Added to these motivations were ones that were more philosophical, sociological, and political. Unless one subscribed to the biomedicalized metabolic theory of addiction underlying the Dole–Nyswander program, the contradictions inherent in treating opioid addiction with an opioid were obvious. In the way that simplistic analogies rarely do much to illuminate the nuance of a controversy, opponents argued that methadone maintenance made as much sense as providing gin to an alcoholic to cure him of his compulsive use of whisky. Since at least the 1920s, theories of addiction ranged in emphasis from deviance and mental illness to sociological conditions of deprivation, but few if any conceived of rehabilitation as implying anything but abstinence.

For many Americans, the issue was a moral one. Yet for others, the questions methadone raised were social and psychological. If one believed, as did most social psychologists, sociologists, and even many psychiatrists, that the "true causes" of addiction—be they social (economic deprivation, denied opportunity, official neglect, racism) or individual (ennui, low self-esteem, anxiety, trauma, depression)—lay in one's psychic engagement with the social world, then methadone did nothing at all to address the problem. Furthermore, the metabolic theory of addiction, comparing it to diabetes, may have been a useful heuristic or analogy to offer politicians and the general public, but it, too, was demonstrably imprecise and simplistic. Few physicians could point to patients who had been able to manage their diabetes to the point where insulin was unnecessary, but stories of successful recovery from even hard-core addiction were easily found, even if not as prodigiously as everyone would have wanted.

It is one thing to believe that heroin addiction among America's youth came from ennui, or lack of meaningful work and purpose, or alienation, or, as in the case of Black and Latino Americans, structural racism. It is something almost completely different to argue that it reflected biological deficiencies in the human body. Black political leadership and racial liberals of all ethnicities generally saw heroin addiction as the result of failed economic policies that had left Black communities without viable jobs, a decent education, secure housing, appropriate health care, and effective public safety. Absent these basic rights, America's Black youth were susceptible to heroin experimentation and addiction. This certainly was a theme embedded in three of the late civil rights-era's most popular memoirs, Claude Brown's *Manchild in the Promised Land* (1965), Alex Haley's and Malcolm X's *The Autobiography of Malcolm X* (1965), and Piri Thomas's *Down These Mean Streets* (1967). If addiction was the direct result of these persisting inequities, any proposal for the provision of a narcotic to narcotics addicts would meet the rejoinder that government officials wanted merely to pacify the ghetto, not to address the deep structural problems that produced addiction. Coined in 1944, the term "genocide" found its way into the political lexicons of a global array of racialized protest movements, and in the

United States framed some of the opposition's analysis of methadone policy among the Black poor.[12]

The medical framing of addiction as a "metabolic disorder" (as Vincent Dole frequently described it), and methadone maintenance for the addicted as analogous to insulin for the diabetic, is one of the 20th century's most pronounced examples of what sociologist Peter Conrad critically called *medicalization*.[13] Indeed, in offering his earliest definition of medicalization—the process of "defining [a specific] behavior as a medical problem or illness and mandating or licensing the medical profession to provide some type of treatment for it"— Conrad listed as examples "alcoholism, drug addiction, and treating violence as a genetic or brain disorder."[14] That all three were behavioral in nature pointed to the historical moment in which Conrad developed the concept. By the early 1970s, medical skepticism, like distrust of all authority, especially government, was at its height. One facet of this was the international antipsychiatry movement, which, somewhat ironically, was led largely by psychiatrists from the United Kingdom, the United States, France, and Italy. In reframing a "deviant" behavior as instead a medical condition, the process of medicalization, so the critique goes, offers the liberation of the individual from social stigma. It also, however, has the potential to turn dynamics that are imminently *social* into *individual pathologies*. Thus they are denunciations of methadone as a "false cure" and an expedient and cheap "technological fix" for issues that government policy had failed to resolve.[15] Psychiatrist Thomas Szasz, one of the most polemical figures in the American antipsychiatry movement, likened the combined carceral and medical authority brought to bear on drug users to the Spanish Inquisition, and methadone to "the Medical Holy Water" designed "to counteract the Heretical Witch's Brew of Heroin."[16] Writing in the journal *Science*, three psychiatrists argued, "If heroin use were 'the problem,' then methadone might well be the answer. If, however, physical, psychological, and social costs of drug use for the person and the community are 'the problem,' then methadone may well contribute to the problem rather than to the solution."[17] Coupled with this logical challenge was the widespread suspicion of what social critics of the time called the "medical–industrial

---

[12] See, for example, Daniel Casriel and Thomas Bratter, "Methadone Maintenance: A Questionable Procedure," *Journal of Drug Issues* 4 (1974); "Methadone a Form of Genocide: Ex-Addict," *New York Amsterdam News*, 10 May 1969; Rev. Curtis E. Burrell Jr., "Black Addiction: A Summary and Overview," *Chicago Daily Defender*, 21 October 1971; William L. Claiborne, "U.S. Methadone Role Scored," *The Washington Post*, 14 May 1972; Audrey Weaver, "From the Weaver," *Chicago Daily Defender*, 29 April 1972; Profumo Adolfo, "Too Many Methadone Clinics = Genocide?," *New York Amsterdam News* 1992; Frank Morales, "Methadone: Genocide of the Poor," *The Portable Lower East Side* 1992.

[13] Peter Conrad, "The Discovery of Hyperkinesis: Notes on the Medicalization of Deviant Behavior," *Social Problems* 23, no. 1 (1975); *Identifying Hyperactive Children : The Medicalization of Deviant Behavior* (Lexington, MA: Lexington Books, 1976); "Medicalization and Social Control," *Annual Review of Sociology* 18 (1992); *Medicalizations*," (United States: American Society for the Advancement of Science, 1992); *Medicalization of Society: On the Transformation of Human Conditions into Treatable Disorders* (United States: The Johns Hopkins University Press, 2007); Peter Conrad and Joseph W. Schneider, "Deviance and Medicalization, from Badness to Sickness," in *Deviance and Medicalization, from Badness to Sickness* (1980).

[14] Conrad, "The Discovery of Hyperkinesis: Notes on the Medicalization of Deviant Behavior."

[15] Dorothy Nelkin, *Methadone Maintenance: A Technological Fix* (New York: G. Braziller, 1973).

[16] Thomas Szasz, *Ceremonial Chemistry: The Ritual Persecution of Drugs, Addicts, and Pushers* (Garden City, NY: Anchor Press, 1974), 67.

[17] Lennard, Epstein, and Rosenthal, "The Methadone Illusion."

complex."[18] This position was exemplified by social scientist Florence Heyman's description in 1972 of methadone as "a typically American answer to a large-scale American problem," and her prediction that rapid and vast proliferation of methadone clinics augured the emergence of a new "bureaucratic empire."[19] At a time when distrust of the government was even more widespread than distrust of organized medicine, many feared a partnership of the two in the form of a methadone empire with an outsized capacity for social control and urban pacification.

The matter of methadone and the variety of medicalization it represented were rendered even more contentious by methadone's place in American anticrime politics and the U.S. history of racialized drug politics and law enforcement. For their own reasons, politicians, journalists, physicians, and social scientists since Emancipation frequently described Black Americans as particularly intemperate and prone to insanity and criminal activity. In the turn of the 20th-century cocaine scare, for example, as drug historian David Musto has observed, "the fear of the cocainized black coincided with the peak of lynchings, legal segregation, and voting laws all designed to remove political and social power from him."[20] In considering the war on crime's origins in the 1960s and 1970s, political scientists Naomi Murakawa and Vesla Weaver and legal scholar Michelle Alexander have argued that anticrime policies, especially the War on Drugs, emerged as a counter to civil rights demands.[21] Speaking specifically of drug law enforcement in the 1950s and 1960s, historian Kathleen Frydl has noted that "African American civil rights leaders had to contend with another discursive construct of the decade, that of [B]lack criminality." Indeed, Senators and Representatives repeatedly highlighted Washington, DC, the nation's only majority Black city, as particularly crime- and drug-ridden. Those who were resistant to the civil rights movement, Frydl also notes, vigorously made "assertions of [B]lack criminality," which they "deployed regularly to counter or to stall the [B]lack freedom movement."[22]

Cognizant of the long history of the popular White association of Black Americans with crime and deviant behavior, and suspicious of methadone maintenance as a convenient technological fix to inconveniently complex social problems, many White and Black Americans therefore wondered which aspect of methadone—addiction recovery or crime reduction—was most attractive to its proponents. The suspicion was not unwarranted. New York's City Council, for example, attempted to pass a bill requiring MMT for as many as 5,000 drug users at Rikers Island jail. Vocal opposition from the City's Commissioners of Corrections, Addiction Services, and Health Services did not deter the largely Democratic council, and it was the veto of Liberal Republican Mayor John Lindsay which ultimately prevented it from becoming law.. New York Governor Nelson Rockefeller's support for methadone programs throughout the state came after

---

[18] Barbara Ehrenreich, John Ehrenreich, and Health/PAC, *The American Health Empire: Power, Profits, and Politics* (New York: Random House, 1970).

[19] Florence Heyman, "Methadone Maintenance as Law and Order," *Society* 9, no. 8 (1972).

[20] David F. Musto, *The American Disease: Origins of Narcotic Control*, 3rd ed. (New York: Oxford University Press, 1999), 7.

[21] Michelle Alexander, *The New Jim Crow: Mass Incarceration in the Age of Colorblindness* (New York: New Presshans, 2010); Vesla M. Weaver, "Frontlash: Race and the Development of Punitive Crime Policy," *Studies in American Political Development* 21, no. 2 (2007); Naomi Murakawa, *The First Civil Right: How Liberals Built Prison America* (New York: Oxford University Press, 2014); Elizabeth Kai Hinton, *From the War on Poverty to the War on Crime : The Making of Mass Incarceration in America* (2016).

[22] Kathleen Frydl, *The Drug Wars in America, 1940-1973* (New York: Cambridge University Press, 2012), 122, 211.

the political and therapeutic disaster of his coercive 1967 civil commitment program, and just before the draconian 1973 drug law, which also bore his name.[23]

Officials at the federal level also expressed enthusiasm for methadone's potential crime-reductive capacities. The 1969 report of the National Commission on the Causes and Prevention of Violence gave significant space to the perceived connections between narcotic addiction and non-violent as well as violent crime, recommending that "more and better [treatment] facilities be established and that research and testing of treatment programs receive high priority [and that] additional research on drug maintenance programs, such as the methadone program in New York, should be encouraged."[24] Federal lawmakers and White House officials closely watched Washington, DC's, crime wave, which had begun in 1966. A February 1969 meeting of Washington's mayor, health department director, and forty other federal and local authorities produced the announcement that the District soon would develop its own methadone program. An influential development had been Vincent Dole's testimony that his program had proven its ability to change hard-core users "from criminals to respectable members of the society."[25] At the 1970 congressional hearings on crime in Washington, DC, even the Superintendent of the U.S. Public Health Service, Dr. Stephen Brown, contended, "we must be honest with ourselves in facing the fact that certainly one of the major things that concern us with opiate addiction is the crime which results from opiate addiction... . It is precisely this criminal activity which would come to an end if heroin addicts... could obtain legal narcotics, such as methadone, from a medically capable source of supply."[26]

Indeed, President Nixon's "therapeutic presidency " (as one historian has called it) was but one side of a Janus-faced drug policy which otherwise emphasized his "War on Drugs" (declared in 1971) and escalated funding and powers directed toward law enforcement efforts.[27] Drug use had not been particularly high on the American public's mind in 1968 – certainly not as worrisome as the economy or the war in Southeast Asia – but Nixon had successfully bundled it into his appeal to conservative white voters whom he termed the "silent majority," and his leadership in skepticism and even outright resistance to peace movements, civil rights activism, gender and reproductive gains, and economic democracy.[28] Commenters at the time noted as much, and there certainly is evidence that Nixon's support for methadone, like his appeal to the silent majority and his "Southern Strategy," was an electoral gambit. Looking ahead to the next election, a 1970 internal White House Domestic Council Summary Option Paper argued that "in 1972 citizens will be looking at crime statistics across the nation in order to see whether expectations raised in 1968 have been met. The federal government has only one economical and

---

[23] Bennett, "Mandated Use of Methadone Assailed by 3 Big City Officials."; Hansen and Roberts, "Two Tiers of Biomedicalization: Buprenorphine, Methadone and the Biopolitics of Addiction Stigma and Race."; Fried, "State Panel Urges Care on Methadone."

[24] Donald J. Mulvihill et al., *Crimes of Violence: A Staff Report Submitted to the National Commission on the Causes & Prevention of Violence*, 3 vols. (Washington, DC: Government Printing Office, 1969).

[25] Philip D. Carter, "City Test of Cheap Drug Set for Heroin Addicts," *Washington Post*, 13 February 1969.

[26] *Crime in the National Capital. Part 2: Narcotics-Crime Crisis in the Washington Area. Hearings before the United States Senate Committee on the District of Columbia*, 1, 25-26 March, and 9-11 April, 1969 1969.

[27] Kevin Yuill, "Another Take on the Nixon Presidency: The First Therapeutic President?," *Journal of Policy History* 21, no. 02 (2009).

[28] David F. Musto and Pamela Korsmeyer, *The Quest for Drug Control: Politics and Federal Policy in a Period of Increasing Substance Abuse, 1963-1981* (New Haven: Yale University Press, 2002).

effective technique for reducing crime in the streets—methadone maintenance."[29] Along with this was the administration's support of measures which were decidedly untherapeutic. In its continuing conflict with the Department of Health, Education, and Welfare regarding authority over the drug use issue, the Department of Justice and its Bureau of Narcotics and Dangerous Drugs seemed to have the support of the President and many influential senators and members of Congress on both sides of the aisle. This imbalance of power gave Justice the authority, provided by the passage of the Comprehensive Drug Abuse Prevention and Control Act of 1970, to perform "no-knock" raids on private residences. That act and the Narcotic Addict Treatment Act of 1974 also made the BNDD's successor, the Drug Enforcement Administration, an equal partner with the FDA in the federal effort to control methadone treatment programs.[30]

There were in fact aspects of the Nixon administration that hailed the first However, many suspected that was not unconnected from his appeal on November 3, 1969, to the "silent majority" of (white, conservative) Americans who had become weary, even resentful, of the politics of antiwar mobilizations, civil rights, gender equality, and economic rights, and distrustful of the post-1933 alliance among organized labor, civil rights, and the Democratic Party.[31]

Many who were following the politics of heroin addiction and methadone understandably expressed concern at the potential abuses of the new treatment modality, and whether massive funding simply tempered a wider agenda of racial control.[32] *Washington Post* columnist William Raspberry opined that "methadone is not so much a means for treating addicts as a way of fighting crime" whose effectiveness in crime reduction would obviate the need for actual treatment from "psychiatrists, social workers, placement specialists and the rest."[33] In two days of hearings on methadone maintenance, U.S. House of Representatives Delegate Walter E. Fauntroy (District of Columbia) made clear his own distrust. So, too, did invited witness Ron Clark, the director of Washington, DC's, RAP, Inc., who argued that MMT was not particularly

---

[29] Quoted in David J. Bellis, *Heroin and Politicians: The Failure of Public Policy to Control Addiction in America*, Contributions in Political Science, (Westport, CT: Greenwood Press, 1981), 59. See also Michael Massing, *The Fix* (New York: Simon & Schuster, 1998).

[30] United States General Accounting Office, *More Effective Action Needed to Control Abuse and Diversion in Methadone Treatment Programs : Food and Drug Administration, Department of Health, Education, and Welfare, Drug Enforcement Administration, Department of Justice : Report to the Congress* (1976).

[31] Mical Raz, "Treating Addiction or Reducing Crime? Methadone Maintenance and Drug Policy under the Nixon Administration," ibid.29, no. 1 (2017); Hinton, *From the War on Poverty to the War on Crime : The Making of Mass Incarceration in America*; Rick Perlstein, *Nixonland: The Rise of a President and the Fracturing of America* (New York: Scribner, 2008); Michael Flamm, "Politics and Pragmatism: The Nixon Administration and Crime Control," *White House Studies* 6, no. 2 (2006); Jason Edwin Glenn, "Medicalizing Addictions, Criminalizing Addicts: Race, Politics and Profit in Narratives of Addiction" (doctoral dissertation, Harvard University, 2005); Ted Galen Carpenter, *Bad Neighbor Policy : Washington's Futile War on Drugs in Latin America*, 1st ed. (New York: Palgrave Macmillan, 2003); Musto and Korsmeyer, *The Quest for Drug Control: Politics and Federal Policy in a Period of Increasing Substance Abuse, 1963-1981*; Dan Baum, *Smoke and Mirrors: The War on Drugs and the Politics of Failure*, 1st ed. (Boston: Little, Brown, 1996); Brooks Jackson, "Nixon Action Aids Capital's Crime Battle," *Los Angeles Times*, 18 November 1971.

[32] Hansen and Roberts, "Two Tiers of Biomedicalization: Buprenorphine, Methadone and the Biopolitics of Addiction Stigma and Race."

[33] William Raspberry, "Holdups or Hangups?," *The Washington Post*, 25 June 1971; "Methadone Use: Another Blunder," *The Washington Post*, 11 May 1971.

beneficial to Black patients or Black communities, but was "politically expedient," for politicians more concerned about crime than recovery."[34]

Historical Lessons

It is tempting to attribute the methadone controversy to mere misunderstanding of the problem and of the other side's perspectives and approaches. It is clear that proponents and opponents, respectively, harbored differing views on the "true causes" and the nature and proper treatment of addiction. By 1970, many of the "drug free" (non-methadone) programs and therapeutic communities based in Black communities connected the heroin problem to official neglect, and addiction treatment to community reconstruction. Though there were some Black methadone doctors in the early years who also connected their work with a larger address of the social structures that, they believed, produced addiction, most methadone physicians were White and by and large exhibited little evidence of doing the same, at least not in ways recognizable to their detractors. Furthermore, their view of their critics and competitors in the addiction treatment marketplace was often uncharitable, even derisive: they regarded the drug-free programs as at best dangerously misguided and, at worst, cynically manipulative. Indeed, in many cases this was true — some programs were based on theories of treatment, which made the programs ineffective, abusive in their tactics, and even cultish. Others, however, were well-run and valued institutions within the communities they served. Meanwhile, leaders of the community-based programs often maintained a caricaturist perception of methadone maintenance as being simply and only the delivery of narcotics to people with addictions. Certainly, many clinics lacked effective supportive services, but rather than critique individual clinics, methadone's most vociferous critics roundly condemned the whole treatment modality.

In fact, the problem was less a misunderstanding than a polarization of opinion as the late 1960s turned into the 1970s. Indeed, we might even posit historical hypotheticals that would illuminate options not taken. First, methadone maintenance represents but one particular form of medicalization of the addiction problem. Alternatively, one might imagine a form of medicalization in a different configuration. Largely because of fear of street diversion, the regulatory view of methadone as a dangerous drug to be heavily regulated effectively shut out the community-based groups who might have used it productively. Indeed, before the stringent regulations of the 1970s, many community-based programs in the 1960s had used methadone informally as a detoxification tool, dispensed every day in gradually decreasing doses. After methadone was taken out of their hands, two of these—the historic programs at Lincoln Detox in the South Bronx and the Blackman's Development Corporation in Washington, DC—were uncompromising in their opposition to methadone maintenance. It is true that there is a great difference between methadone detoxification and methadone maintenance, but this historical example shows that these groups were not categorically against the use of a narcotic on the way to recovery.

It is certainly imaginable that there could have been a methadone maintenance system more closely aligned with the community mental health and free clinic movements. These movements thrived during the War on Poverty years, but fell out of federal favor after 1969. In regard to methadone, in 1970 and after, federal policy was primarily concerned with keeping methadone out of the wrong hands, and less interested in ensuring that it was in the right ones. In

---

[34] Peter Osnos, "Is It a Solution?: Controversy on Methadone as Heroin Solution Mounting," ibid., 26 December 1972.

a different but imaginable policy environment (one in which the federal government had maintained its commitment to the Great Society, one in which BNDD and DEA power did not so dramatically outmatch the influence of physicians and community-based groups), federal policy might have provided compelling incentives to methadone physicians to partner with or to lodge their practices within the local organizations that had better connections to the communities they served. A feature of nearly all of the spectrum of Black political thought, the political investment in addiction rehabilitation as community building, did not preclude the daily use of a substance in the service of positive psychic and social change. Had policy makers thought it a worthwhile policy experiment, the deliberate coupling of methadone with the therapeutic communities might have helped to reduce stigma. No such policy was ever explored, but a great deal of effort and resources were expended in policing methadone physicians in the name of preventing their inventories from being diverted to the street.

These notions are counterfactual, but not inconceivable. Indeed, some could have come to be as a matter of historical accident. However, one factor is difficult to imagine as being any different except outside of the United States' longer history of anti-Black racism and stigma against people who use substances. To speculate about what might have or might have not happened under a different presidential administration, or within a different regulatory structure, is relatively simple compared with the exercise of imagining how methadone maintenance might have emerged without the 350 years of history which preceded it. This consideration, however, is perhaps the most important in future drug policy. After all, heroin and virtually all of the drugs popularly described as "dangerous" in U.S. history were deeply racialized in politics and the policy arena. The War on Drugs, announced by President Nixon, but accelerated under Presidents Reagan, Bush, and Clinton, was, as we now understand, a deeply racialized enterprise. Methadone had nothing to say to that, while many social scientists and the highest profile Black drug-free community-based treatment centers took that history as a point of departure for theories of personality development. Many individuals realized successful and meaningful recovery under each approach, but one wonders what might have been had those seeking recovery not been forced to choose one over the other.

To be clear, I do not argue that popular stigma in Black political culture is today the primary barrier to the realization of good treatment. First, Black stigma against methadone may be distinguishable from other Americans' stigmatizing attitudes only in its political nature, not in its prevalence or intensity. Second, compared with structural impediments, stigma is much less "material." At the same time, understanding the nature of Black popular disapproval of methadone is of material concern, as the continued stigmatization of people in medically assisted treatment inevitably will prevent us from seeing them as citizens whose needs are not much different from other groups with specific health care requirements.

Unlike legal protection, educational equity, or economic opportunity, the needs and rights of people who use drugs was not a major plank in any civil rights platform of the 1950s, 1960s, 1970s, and 1980s. None of the movement's national or local leaders made this a priority in their negotiations with power. However, unlike 50-plus years ago, today we have the benefit of a widely distributed network of Black harm reductionists, many of whom began their work in the 1980s and whose principal agenda combines, among other things, accessibility to health care and a frontal attack on stigma. An imaginable future of therapeutic success certainly must include the peer counselors, volunteers, policy workers, and physicians who comprise this 21st century movement for civil and human rights.

WORKS CITED

Adolfo, Profumo. "Too Many Methadone Clinics = Genocide?" *New York Amsterdam News*, 1992, 13.

Alexander, Michelle. *The New Jim Crow: Mass Incarceration in the Age of Colorblindness.* New York: New Press, 2010.

Allen, Bennett, Michelle L. Nolan, and Denise Paone. "Underutilization of Medications to Treat Opioid Use Disorder: What Role Does Stigma Play?". *Substance Abuse* 40, no. 4 (2019/10/02 2019): 459-65.

Andraka-Christou, Barbara. "Addressing Racial and Ethnic Disparities in the Use of Medications for Opioid Use Disorder.". *Health Affairs* 40, no. 6 (2021): 920-27.

Baum, Dan. *Smoke and Mirrors: The War on Drugs and the Politics of Failure.* 1st ed. Boston: Little, Brown, 1996.

Bellis, David J. *Heroin and Politicians: The Failure of Public Policy to Control Addiction in America.* Contributions in Political Science. Westport, CT: Greenwood Press, 1981.

Bennett, Charles G. "Mandated Use of Methadone Assailed by 3 Big City Officials." *New York Times*, 8 February 1969, 32.

Burrell Jr., Rev. Curtis E. "Black Addiction: A Summary and Overview." *Chicago Daily Defender*, 21 October 1971.

Carpenter, Ted Galen. *Bad Neighbor Policy: Washington's Futile War on Drugs in Latin America.* 1st ed. New York: Palgrave Macmillan, 2003.

Carter, Philip D. "City Test of Cheap Drug Set for Heroin Addicts." *Washington Post*, 13 February 1969, A1.

Casriel, Daniel, and Thomas Bratter. "Methadone Maintenance: A Questionable Procedure." *Journal of Drug Issues* 4 (1974): 359-75.

Claiborne, William L. "U.S. Methadone Role Scored." *The Washington Post*, 14 May 1972, D1.

"Clergymen Back, Hit Giving Dope to Addicts." *New York Amsterdam News* 22 February 1964, 20.

"Conditions for Investigational Use of Methadone for Maintenance Programs for Narcotic Addicts." *Federal Register* 35, no. 113 (11 June 1970): 9014-16.

Conner, Kyaien O., and Daniel Rosen. "'You're Nothing but a Junkie': Multiple Experiences of Stigma in an Aging Methadone Maintenance Population." *Journal of Social Work Practice in the Addictions* 8, no. 2 (2008): 244-64.

Conner, Kyaien O., Daniel Rosen, Sandra Wexle, and Charlotte Brown. "It's Like Night and Day. He's White. I'm Black: Shared Stigmas between Counselors and Older Adult Methadone Clients." *Best Practices in Mental Health* 6, no. 1 (January 2010): 17-32.

Conrad, Peter. "The Discovery of Hyperkinesis: Notes on the Medicalization of Deviant Behavior." *Social Problems* 23, no. 1 (1975): 12-21.

———. *Identifying Hyperactive Children: The Medicalization of Deviant Behavior.* Lexington, MA: Lexington Books, 1976.

———. "Medicalization and Social Control." *Annual Review of Sociology* 18 (1992): 209-32.

———. *Medicalization of Society: On the Transformation of Human Conditions into Treatable Disorders.* United States: The Johns Hopkins University Press, 2007.

———. "Medicalizations." 334-35. United States: American Society for the Advancement of

APPENDIX C

Science, 1992.
Conrad, Peter, and Joseph W. Schneider. "Deviance and Medicalization, from Badness to Sickness." In *Deviance and Medicalization, from Badness to Sickness*, 1980.
Courtwright, David, Herman Joseph, and Don Des Jarlais. *Addicts Who Survived: An Oral History of Narcotic Use in America, 1923-1965*. Knoxville: University of Tennessee Press, 1989.
Crime in the National Capital. Part 2: Narcotics–Crime Crisis in the Washington Area. Hearings before the United States Senate Committee on the District of Columbia, 1, 25-26 March, and 9-11 April, 1969.
Ehrenreich, Barbara, John Ehrenreich, and Health/PAC. *The American Health Empire: Power, Profits, and Politics*. New York: Random House, 1970.
Flamm, Michael. "Politics and Pragmatism: The Nixon Administration and Crime Control." *White House Studies* 6, no. 2 (2006): 151-62.
Fried, Joseph P. "State Panel Urges Care on Methadone." *New York Times*, 17 May 1969, 34.
Frydl, Kathleen. *The Drug Wars in America, 1940-1973*. New York: Cambridge University Press, 2012.
Glenn, Jason Edwin. "Medicalizing Addictions, Criminalizing Addicts: Race, Politics and Profit in Narratives of Addiction." Doctoral dissertation, Harvard University, 2005.
Hagle, Holly N., Marlene Martin, Rachel Winograd, Jessica Merlin, Deborah S. Finnell, Jeffrey P. Bratberg, Adam J. Gordon, *et al.* "Dismantling Racism against Black, Indigenous, and People of Color across the Substance Use Continuum: A Position Statement of the Association for Multidisciplinary Education and Research in Substance Use and Addiction." [In English]. *Substance abuse* 42, no. 1 (2021): 5-12.
Height, Dorothy. "A Woman's Word." *New York Amsterdam News*, 4 September 1965, 34.
Heyman, Florence. "Methadone Maintenance as Law and Order." *Society* 9, no. 8 (June 1972): 15-25.
Hilts, Philip J. *Protecting America's Health: The FDA, Business, and One Hundred Years of Regulation*. New York: Alfred A. Knopf, 2003.
Hinton, Elizabeth Kai. *From the War on Poverty to the War on Crime: The Making of Mass Incarceration in America*. 2016.
Hudgins, Anastasia, Beth Uzwiak, Lia Pizzicato, and Kendra Viner. "Barriers to Effective Care: Specialty Drug Treatment in Philadelphia." [In English]. *Journal of substance abuse treatment* 131 (2021): 108639-39.
Jackson, Brooks. "Nixon Action Aids Capital's Crime Battle." *Los Angeles Times*, 18 November 1971, B4, B5.
King, Joseph P., Lonnie MacDonald, and Harlem Neighborhoods Association Inc. (HANA). "A Preliminary Report of the Neighborhood Conference on Narcotics Addiction, Co-Sponsored by Harlem Neighborhoods Association Mental Health Committee, Harlem Hospital Department of Psychiatry." Malcolm X Papers, Schomburg Center for Black History and Culture; Box 10, Folder 14, 1963.
Knight, Kelly Ray. *Addicted.Pregnant.Poor*. Durham, NC: Duke University Press, 2015.
Lennard, Henry L., Leon J. Epstein, and Mitchell S. Rosenthal. "The Methadone Illusion." *Science* 176, no. 4037 (26 May 1972): 881-84.
Massing, Michael. *The Fix*. New York: Simon & Schuster, 1998.
"Methadone a Form of Genocide: Ex-Addict." *New York Amsterdam News*, 10 May 1969, 37.
"Methadone Plans Called Unworkable." *The Austin Statesman*, 13 July 1970, 29.

Methadone Use and Abuse -- 1972-73. Hearings before the Subcommittee to Investigate Juvenile Delinquency of the Senate Committee on the Judiciary; November 14 and 16, 1972; February 8, 13, and 14, 1973 and April 6, 1973, Second Session of the 92nd Congress and First Session of the 93rd Congress, 1973.

Morales, Frank. "Methadone: Genocide of the Poor." *The Portable Lower East Side*, 1992, 107-12.

Mulvihill, Donald J., Melvin M. Tumin, Lynn A. Curtis, United States Task Force on Individual Acts of Violence, and United States National Commission on the Causes and Prevention of Violence. *Crimes of Violence: A Staff Report Submitted to the National Commission on the Causes & Prevention of Violence*. 3 vols. Washington, DC: Government Printing Office, 1969.

Murakawa, Naomi. *The First Civil Right: How Liberals Built Prison America*. New York: Oxford University Press, 2014.

Musto, David F. *The American Disease: Origins of Narcotic Control*. 3rd ed. New York: Oxford University Press, 1999.

Musto, David F., and Pamela Korsmeyer. *The Quest for Drug Control: Politics and Federal Policy in a Period of Increasing Substance Abuse, 1963-1981*. New Haven: Yale University Press, 2002.

Nelkin, Dorothy. *Methadone Maintenance: A Technological Fix*. New York: G. Braziller, 1973.

Osnos, Peter. "Is It a Solution?: Controversy on Methadone as Heroin Solution Mounting." *The Washington Post*, 26 December 1972.

Perlstein, Rick. *Nixonland: The Rise of a President and the Fracturing of America*. New York: Scribner, 2008.

Raspberry, William. "Holdups or Hangups?" *The Washington Post*, 25 June 1971.

———. "Methadone Use: Another Blunder." *The Washington Post*, 11 May 1971.

Raz, Mical. "Treating Addiction or Reducing Crime? Methadone Maintenance and Drug Policy under the Nixon Administration." *Journal of Policy History* 29, no. 1 (2017): 58-86.

Saloner, Brendan, Emma E. McGinty, Leo Beletsky, Ricky Bluthenthal, Chris Beyrer, Michael Botticelli, and Susan G. Sherman. "A Public Health Strategy for the Opioid Crisis." [In English]. *Public health reports (1974)* 133, no. 1S (2018): 24S-34S.

"Should Dope Be Legalized? Doctors, Police and Social Workers Debate Drastic Move to Set up Legal Clinics as Step to Combat Narcotics Racket." *Ebony Magazine*, April 1953, 88-94.

Szasz, Thomas. *Ceremonial Chemistry: The Ritual Persecution of Drugs, Addicts, and Pushers*. Garden City, NY: Anchor Press, 1974.

Tsai, Alexander C., Mathew V. Kiang, Michael L. Barnett, Leo Beletsky, Katherine M. Keyes, Emma E. McGinty, Laramie R. Smith, et al. "Stigma as a Fundamental Hindrance to the United States Opioid Overdose Crisis Response." [In English]. *PLoS medicine* 16, no. 11 (2019): e1002969-e69.

United States Food and Drug Administration. "Proposed Rules, Department of Health, Education, and Welfare. Food and Drug Administration Conditions for Investigational Use of Methadone for Maintenance Programs for Narcotic Addicts." *Federal Register* 35, no. 113 (11 June 1970): 9000-01, 14-15.

United States General Accounting Office. *More Effective Action Needed to Control Abuse and Diversion in Methadone Treatment Programs: Food and Drug Administration, Department of Health, Education, and Welfare, Drug Enforcement Administration, Department of Justice: Report to the Congress*. 1976.

APPENDIX C

Walters, Ida. "Curse or Cure?" *Wall Street Journal*, 27 July 1972, 1.
Weaver, Audrey. "From the Weaver." *Chicago Daily Defender*, 29 April 1972.
Weaver, Vesla M. "Frontlash: Race and the Development of Punitive Crime Policy." *Studies in American Political Development* 21, no. 2 (2007): 230-65.
Witte, Tricia H., Jessica Jaiswal, Mercy N. Mumba, and George C. T. Mugoya. "Stigma Surrounding the Use of Medically Assisted Treatment for Opioid Use Disorder." *Substance Use & Misuse* 56, no. 10 (2021/08/24 2021): 1467-75.
Wolfson, Lindsay, Rose A. Schmidt, Julie Stinson, and Nancy Poole. "Examining Barriers to Harm Reduction and Child Welfare Services for Pregnant Women and Mothers Who Use Substances Using a Stigma Action Framework." [In English]. *Health & social care in the community* 29, no. 3 (2021): 589-601.
Woo, Julia, Anuja Bhalerao, Monica Bawor, Meha Bhatt, Brittany Dennis, Natalia Mouravska, Laura Zielinski, and Zainab Samaan. "'Don't Judge a Book by Its Cover': A Qualitative Study of Methadone Patients' Experiences of Stigma." *Substance Abuse: Research and Treatment* 11 (2017).
Yuill, Kevin. "Another Take on the Nixon Presidency: The First Therapeutic President?". *Journal of Policy History* 21, no. 02 (2009): 138-62.

Federal Administrative Pathways to Promote Access to Quality Methadone Treatment

February 21, 2022

Matthew B. Lawrence[*]

Emory University School of Law

Synopsis

The National Academies of Science, Engineering, and Medicine commissioned this paper for *Methadone Treatment for Opioid Use Disorder: Examining Federal Regulations and Laws – A Workshop*. It surveys pathways through which federal agencies could promote access to quality methadone treatment by utilizing existing legal authorities, without the need for federal or state legislation. It reviews existing analyses identifying specific pathways that federal agencies already have authority to utilize and points to promising areas in which further research may reveal additional flexibilities. Topic areas include the Substance Abuse and Mental Health Services Administration's (SAMHSA) standard-setting and Drug Enforcement Administration's (DEA) waiver authorities under the Controlled Substances Act; Health and Human Services Office of Inspector General (HHS OIG) authorities related to the antikickback statute; statutory and constitutional checks on state and opioid treatment program (OTP) restrictions; and payment authorities related to Medicare, Medicaid, and employer-sponsored insurance.

---

[*] The author is responsible for the content of this article, which does not necessarily represent the views of the National Academies of Sciences, Engineering, and Medicine.

Federal Administrative Pathways to Promote Access to Quality Methadone Treatment

Table of Contents

Introduction 153
I. Controlled Substances Act 154
    A. Dispensing 154
    B. Distribution 154
    C. Quality 155
II. Antikickback Statute and Civil Monetary Penalties Statute 155
III. State Restrictions 156
IV. Payment 156
    A. Traditional Medicare 156
    B. Medicare Advantage 157
    C. Medicaid 158
    D. Employer-Sponsored Insurance 159
Conclusion 159

Introduction

A 2019 National Academies Report explained that although methadone is an effective treatment for opioid use disorder, significant and inequitable barriers impede access.[1] This paper surveys possible pathways through which federal administrative agencies could overcome or mitigate some barriers to quality methadone treatment, without the need for legislation. It builds on prior literature either establishing (as legally permissible) or exploring (as worthy of further consideration) such pathways.[2] The paper does not necessarily endorse utilization of the pathways it identifies, but simply notes their availability or potential availability.

Agencies have two main ways to effectuate legal change without legislation. Statutes often give agencies broad authority over implementation. Where current legal requirements stem from regulation, they can usually be changed through notice-and-comment rulemaking so long as the new rules remain within the underlying statutory mandate. In other cases, agencies are charged with enforcing statutes, regulations,

---

[1] NATIONAL ACADS. OF SCIENCES, ENGINEERING, AND MED., MEDICATIONS FOR OPIOID USE DISORDER SAVE LIVES at 9-10 (2019).
[2] Bridget C.E. Dooling & Laura Stanley, *Extending Pandemic Flexibilities for Opioid Use Disorder Treatment: Unsupervised Use of Opioid Treatment Medications*, 105 MINN. L. REV. HEADNOTES 74 (2021); Corey S. Davis and Derek H. Carr, *Legal and policy changes urgently needed to increase access to opioid agonist therapy in the United States*, 73 INT. J. DRUG POL'Y 42-48 (2019).

or even constitutional provisions. Enforcement policy can ordinarily be changed by the agency without rulemaking.

I. Controlled Substances Act

A. Dispensing

Section 823(g) of the Controlled Substances Act (CSA) requires "practitioners who dispense narcotic drugs" for maintenance of detoxification treatment to obtain an annual registration.[37] It also provides that registrations should be granted only to practitioners who meet standards "established by [SAMHSA]" governing practitioner qualifications, the security of narcotics, and their provision for unsupervised use.[38] The standards established by the Substance Abuse and Mental Health Services Administration (SAMHSA) create the category of "Opioid Treatment Programs (OTPs),"[39] set rules governing OTPs,[40] and provide for accreditation bodies to oversee OTP operations.[41]

Dooling and Stanley point out that CSA "plainly gives SAMHSA broad authority to establish the standards practitioners must follow in order to be registered," which includes the power to change those standards.[42] Davis and Carr also read the statute to grant SAMHSA broad discretion and call for a variety of changes in the current regulatory requirements.[43]

In addition to SAMHSA's standard-setting authority, CSA gives the Drug Enforcement Administration (DEA) authority to "waive the requirement for registration of certain manufacturers, distributors, or dispensers if [DEA] finds it consistent with the public health and safety."[44] DEA recently employed this waiver authority to create mobile van flexibilities.[45]

SAMHSA's standard-setting authority and DEA's waiver authority are promising pathways for administrative adoption of essentially any of the changes in CSA requirements that scholars have proposed. For example, Pytell and colleagues recommend changes "to expressly allow for hospitals to initiate and adjust the dose of methadone."[46] Such reforms could be made through notice and comment rulemaking using either the Secretary's standard-setting authority or the Attorney General's waiver authority.

B. Distribution

---

[37] 21 U.S.C. § 823(g).
[38] *Id.* § 823(g)(2).
[39] 42 C.F.R. § 8.12.
[40] *Id.*
[41] *Id.* § 8.13.
[42] Dooling & Stanley, *supra* note 36 at 12.
[43] Davis & Carr, *supra* note 36.
[44] 21 U.S.C. § 822(d).
[45] 86 Fed. Reg. 33861 (2021); Taleed El-Sabawi et al., *The New Mobile Methadone Rules and What They Mean for Treatment Access*, HEALTH AFFAIRS BLOG, August 4, 2021.
[46] Jarratt D. Pytell et al., *Facilitating Methadone Use in Hospitals and Skilled Nursing Facilities*, 180 JAMA INTERN. MED. 6-7 (2019).

Reports suggest that hospitals and skilled nursing facilities have difficulty obtaining sufficient quantities of methadone to administer to eligible patients.[47] Buprenorphine shortages trace in part to pharmacies' fear that ordering sufficient quantities will place them above an unwritten threshold that triggers DEA investigation.[48] To address this barrier, DEA could clarify in guidance that increasing stocks of methadone to provide to hospitals or skilled nursing facilities will not trigger enforcement consequences.

C. Quality

The Methadone Manifesto describes the withholding of methadone as a form of punishment by some OTPs as a barrier to maintenance of treatment.[49] SAMHSA could potentially use its standard-setting authority to address these concerns. Alternatively, the agency could, through its routine oversight of accreditation bodies, press for greater scrutiny of OTP conduct.[50]

Further research could also explore the possibility of litigation challenging OTP behavior under the Due Process Clause of the U.S. Constitution. Through the "state action doctrine," courts may deem a private actor to be acting as a government actor and subject to constitutional requirements. A thorough analysis of how the complicated legal test for the state action doctrine applies to OTPs in light of their unique role under the CSA would be necessary to determine the viability of this pathway to check OTP behavior.

II. Antikickback Statute and Civil Monetary Penalties Statute

Contingency management is a treatment employing rewards that can be effective for stimulants increasingly used alongside opioids.[51] Take-up of this form of treatment has been limited, however, in part by provider concerns that the provision of rewards to patients may give rise to liability under the federal antikickback statute (AKS) or the civil monetary penalty statute (CMP).[52] Generally speaking, these laws limit offering remuneration to patients unless a safe harbor is present.[53]

The Department of Health and Human Services (HHS) Office of Inspector General (OIG) enforces these statutes and has authority to implement safe harbors. OIG has declined to create a safe harbor for contingency management.[54] This does not mean that contingency management violates the law, but it leaves violation in any individual case a fact-intensive determination that providers may wish to avoid. OIG could mitigate this barrier by using its authority to promulgate safe harbors by regulation,[55] or use its enforcement discretion to describe situations in which contingency management will not be subject to liability.

---

[47] David Gifford et al., *Additional Barriers to Methadone Use in Hospitals and Skilled Nursing Facilities*, 180 JAMA INTERN. MED. 615 (2020).
[48] Hannah Cooper et al., *When Prescribing Isn't Enough—Pharmacy-Level Barriers to Buprenorphine Access*, 383 NEW ENG. J. MED. 703 (2020).
[49] Urban Survivors Union, *Methadone Manifesto* at 29, https://sway.office.com/UjvQx4ZNnXAYxhe7?ref=Link&mc_cid=9754583648&mc_eid=51fa67f051.
[50] *See* HHS OIG, *SAMHSA's Oversight of Accreditation Bodies for Opioid Treatment Programs Did Not Comply with Some Federal Requirements* (A-09-18-01007).
[51] 85 Fed. Reg. 77791 (Dec. 2, 2020).
[52] *Id.*
[53] 42 U.S.C. § 1320a-7b(b); 42 U.S.C. § 1320a-7a(a)(5).
[54] 85 Fed. Reg. 77791 (Dec. 2, 2020); *see also id.* (discussing application of $75 *de minimis* exception).
[55] 42 U.S.C. § 1320a-7b(b)(3)(E).

Furthermore, "incentives offered as part of a CMS-sponsored model may qualify for protection under the safe harbor" for payment models.[56] Thus, the Centers for Medicare & Medicaid Services (CMS) could, by creating or expanding payment models for methadone treatment, render connected contingency management protected from liability under these statutes.

III. State Restrictions

Many states impose restrictions on methadone prescribing that are more stringent than federal requirements.[57] Two pathways to overcome these barriers warrant further consideration. The Department of Justice's Office of Civil Rights, which has reportedly discussed an "Opioid Initiative," may be the best positioned federal agency unit to explore these pathways.

First, because the U.S. Constitution makes federal law the "supreme Law of the Land,"[58] state laws that are inconsistent with federal statutory or regulatory requirements can be "preempted" — rendered void — as a result of that inconsistency.[59] Preemption doctrine is complex,[60] but future research might explore whether there are ways that current or future DEA waivers (e.g., the mobile van waiver), SAMHSA standards, or CMS payment models could be preemptive.

Second, state barriers to methadone treatment may themselves violate federal law or the U.S. Constitution. Friedman and Trent describe several theories on which restrictions on access to methadone in prison or in other institutional settings might run afoul of prohibitions on discrimination against individuals with disabilities in the Americans with Disabilities Act and Rehabilitation Act of 1973.[61] Furthermore, a work in progress by the author concludes there is a reasonable legal argument that unjustified state restrictions on access to methadone implicate a fundamental liberty interest under the Fourteenth Amendment.[62]

IV. Payment

A. Traditional Medicare

Provider participation and patient access are both a function of the generosity of payment.[63] Traditional Medicare now covers OTP services without payer utilization management or cost sharing through a bundled payment model.[64] In 2021 CMS issued an emergency rule to prevent a cut in

---

[56] 85 Fed. Reg. at 77792.
[57] Corey S. Davis & Amy Judd Lieberman, *Access to Treatment for Individuals with Substance Use Disorder* at 115 Covid-19 Policy Playbook (2021) (discussing state barriers).
[58] U.S. CONST. art. VI, cl. 2.
[59] *See generally* Jonathan Nash, *Null Preemption*, 85 NOTRE DAME L. REV. 1015 (2010).
[60] *Id.*
[61] Sally Friedman & Melissa Trent, *Defense Lawyers and the Opioid Epidemic: Advocating for Addiction Medication* at 26, NACDL.Org.
[62] Matthew B. Lawrence, *Addiction and Liberty* (work in progress).
[63] Rebecca L. Haffajee et al., *Policy Pathways to Address Provider Workforce Barriers to Buprenorphine Treatment*, 54 AM. J. PREV. MED. (2018).
[64] *See generally* 84 Fed. Reg. 62673 (Nov. 15, 2019).

reimbursement rates for this bundle for 2022, and the agency is now considering a revision to its formula to ensure appropriate compensation for OTPs in future years.[65] This ongoing administrative proceeding is a ready legal path by which the agency could promote access to methadone.

Additionally, it is unclear how methadone provided through pharmacies, hospitals, or primary care would be paid through the existing Medicare bundled model, so it may be appropriate for CMS to consider offering alternative payment options — including coverage as a preferred drug (like buprenorphine) through Medicare Part D — to promote the financial viability of such reforms.[66] CMS has broad authorities to implement payment reforms through the regulatory process.[67]

B. Medicare Advantage

Medicare Advantage (MA) plans must now cover methadone, but they may currently limit that coverage with cost-sharing requirements for beneficiaries and/or utilization management (including prior authorization, step therapy, and utilization review).[68] Utilization management can be a significant barrier to medication-assisted treatment (MAT),[69] and CMS has indicated that it is "considering strategies . . . to monitor the implementation of the OTP benefit by MA plans . . . including what data might be available to evaluate plan performance."[70]

Two administrative pathways are available to CMS to mitigate the risk that MA plans will impose unjustified barriers through utilization management. First, CMS reviews the adequacy of MA plans' networks at various stages of plan creation and administration to ensure adequate coverage of essential services, including time and distance criteria for 27 provider specialty types.[71] CMS's guidance on the specialties it includes in this review does not currently include OTPs.[72] CMS could update this guidance to include OTP coverage in its assessment of network adequacy.

Second, MA plans are paid through a "risk adjustment" system that mitigates insurers' incentive to impose artificial barriers to treatment for properly adjusted diagnoses.[73] The Affordable Care Act required CMS periodically to "evaluate and revise the [MA] risk adjustment system . . . in order to, as accurately as possible, account for higher medical and care coordination costs associated with . . . a diagnosis of mental illness."[74] CMS has to date failed to meaningfully perform this evaluation and revision, and doing so would offer a pathway to promote access to methadone treatment.[75]

---

[65] 86 Fed. Reg. 66031 (Nov. 19, 2021).
[66] *Cf.* 86 Fed. Reg. 66031-32 ("methadone cannot be dispensed by a pharmacy . . . and therefore is not covered under Medicare Part D").
[67] *E.g.*, § 1115A; 42 U.S.C. § 1395(d)(5)(i)(I).
[68] 84 Fed. Reg. 62762 (Nov. 15, 2019).
[69] Daniel M. Hartung et al., *Buprenorphine Coverage in the Medicare Part D Program for 2007 to 2018*, 321 JAMA 607–609 (2019).
[70] 84 Fed. Reg. at 62762 (Nov. 15, 2019).
[71] CMS, *Medicare Advantage Network Adequacy Criteria Guidance* (Jan. 10, 2017).
[72] 85 Fed. Reg. at 62762.
[73] T. G. McGuire, *Achieving Mental Health Care Parity Might Require Changes in Payments and Competition*, HEALTH AFFAIRS, 35, No. 6 (2016): 1029-1035.
[74] 42 U.S.C. 1395w-23(a)(1)(C)(iii)(III).
[75] Matthew B. Lawrence, *Regulatory Pathways to Promote Treatment for Substance Use Disorder or Other Under-Treated Conditions Using Risk Adjustment*, 46 JLME 935 (2019).

C. Medicaid

Section 1006(b) of the SUPPORT [Substance Use-Disorder Prevention that Promotes Opioid Recovery and Treatment for Patients and Communities] Act required all states to cover methadone through Medicaid. Seventy-five percent of Medicaid enrollees are in a managed care plan that may impose barriers to methadone treatment through unjustified prior authorization, step therapy, annual or lifetime caps, or utilization review requirements.[76]

Federal law restricts coverage limitations in Medicaid to situations where it is medically necessary or needed to prevent waste.[77] CMS has the authority to enforce these requirements,[78] but it is currently difficult for the agency to assess compliance because "[d]ata submitted by managed care plans to states and by states to CMS vary in their consistency, availability, and timeliness."[79] CMS's statutory authority regarding data submissions by managed care plans and states,[80] then, is a promising legal avenue to develop the data necessary for more effective enforcement. By requiring more uniform and comprehensive submission of data regarding utilization management practices, CMS could position itself to assess the scope of inappropriate barriers and enforce or strengthen existing requirements.

More broadly, Medicaid is subject to two major administrative authorities that offer pathways to address social determinants that fuel the epidemic and impede access to treatment.[81] Section 1115 empowers CMS to grant federal matching payments for state costs that are not ordinarily matchable through the program.[82] The statute does not require these payments to be budget neutral.[83] North Carolina has received a waiver under this authority, for example, to pay for housing, transportation, and other supports aimed at the social determinants of health.[84] CMS has issued reports surveying steps that states have taken and might take to support housing for people with substance use disorder through the Medicaid program.[85] For any states interested in addressing social and economic barriers to methadone treatment, section 1115 holds the potential to serve as a significant source of funding and flexibility.

Section 1115A empowers CMS to test innovative payment models within Medicare or Medicaid. It has already developed two such models relevant to methadone, the Maternal Opioid Misuse model[86] and

---

[76] J.V. Jacobi, *The ABCs (Accessibility, Barriers, and Challenges) of Medicaid Expansion: Medicaid, Managed Care, and the Mission for the Poor*, ST. LOUIS UNIV. J. OF HEALTH LAW & POL'Y 9, no. 2 (2016).
[77] 42 U.S.C. § 1396r–8(d); 42 C.F.R. § 440.230; 42 U.S.C. § 1396o-1(c) (addressing preferred drugs).
[78] *See* 42 U.S.C. §§ 1396u–2, 1396n(b), 1315(a).
[79] Medicaid & CHIP Payment & Access Comm'n, *Report to the Congress: The Evolution of Managed Care in Medicaid* 64 (June 2011).
[80] *E.g.*, 42 U.S.C. § 1927(g) (describing drug use review programs).
[81] *See* Nabarun Dasgupta, Leo Beletsky, & Daniel Ciccarone, *Opioid Crisis: No Easy Fix to Its Social and Economic Determinants*, 108 AM. J. PUB. HEALTH 182 (2018) (discussing root causes).
[82] Matthew B. Lawrence, *Fiscal Waivers and State "Innovation" in Health Care*, 62 WM. & MARY L. REV. 123 (2020).
[83] *Id.*
[84] https://www.kff.org/report-section/a-first-look-at-north-carolinas-section-1115-medicaid-waivers-healthy-opportunities-pilots-issue-brief/.
[85] U.S. Department of Health and Human Services, *Report to the President and Congress Section 1018 Action Plan for Technical Assistance and Support for Innovative State Strategies to Provide Housing-Related Supports to Individuals with Substance Use Disorder Under Medicaid* (July 2019).
[86] https://innovation.cms.gov/innovation-models/maternal-opioid-misuse-model.

the Integrated Care for Kids model.[87] Section 1115A could offer a vehicle for administrative adoption of any other payment reforms policy makers deem beneficial.

D. Employer-Sponsored Insurance

Finally, patients who have insurance through an employee benefit plan may also face unjustified barriers to coverage.[88] The Paul Wellstone and Pete Domenici Mental Health Parity and Addiction Equity Act of 2008[89] offers some protection, prohibiting discrimination against mental illness in the design and administration of benefits. The law is administered by the Department of Labor, which recently issued a report noting that "health plans and health insurance issuers are failing to deliver parity for mental health and substance-use disorder benefits to those they cover."[90] For example, one large employer plan with 7,600 beneficiaries excluded coverage for methadone altogether without imposing analogous restrictions on physical health treatments and without the required comparative supporting analysis.[91]

The 2021 Consolidated Appropriations Act gave the Department of Labor new authorities related to the investigation of parity requirements through non-quantified treatment limitations (e.g., prior authorization and medical necessity review),[92] and the agency is now beginning to implement these authorities despite limited resources and enforcement powers.

Conclusion

Significant legal change to promote access to quality methadone treatment could be accomplished without legislation. There are promising pathways toward such change within the authorities of the Department of Health and Human Services (CMS, OIG, and SAMHSA), the Department of Justice (DEA and Office for Civil Rights), and the Department of Labor.

---

[87] https://innovation.cms.gov/innovation-models/integrated-care-for-kids-model.
[88] Daniel Polsky et al., *Private Coverage of Methadone in Outpatient Treatment Programs*. 71 PSYCHIATR. SERV. 303-306 (2020).
[89] Pub. L. No. 100-343 § § 511-12, 122 Stat. 365 (codified at 29 U.S.C. § 1185a & 42 U.S.C. § 300gg-26 (2012)).
[90] https://www.dol.gov/newsroom/releases/ebsa/ebsa20220125.
[91] *Id.*
[92] Section 203, CAA.

Innovations in Methadone Medication for Opioid Use Disorder: A Scoping Review

February 20, 2022

Wes Williams[*]

J.D. Candidate

University of Virginia School of Law

Abstract

Methadone, an opioid agonist, is an effective treatment for opioid use disorder (OUD). Methadone both lowers the likelihood of overdose and reduces illicit opioid use. However, a fairly narrow regulatory approach currently limits methadone access. Methadone currently may be dispensed for the treatment of OUD only in federally approved opioid treatment programs (OTPs).[1] This scoping review identifies and reviews the effects of different approaches to methadone medication for OUD (MOUD) aside from the most common treatment pathway used by OTPs under the current regulatory landscape. The alternatives include modifications allowed in response to the COVID-19 pandemic as well as treatment practices outside the United States. The review identifies multiple ways clinicians have tried to address barriers to access in response to the needs of rural patients or to pandemic obstacles. Early studies of the pandemic response have shown no decrease in quality of treatment or patient outcomes in response to increased take-home dosing and use of telehealth, although telehealth treatment has shown to be less accessible for patients without broadband or smartphone access. Both U.S. and international studies of office-based and pharmacy-based MOUD suggest they present opportunities to increase access to MOUD, especially for rural patients, without worsening treatment outcomes.

INTRODUCTION

Opioid use disorder (OUD) is a chronic brain disease that affects millions of Americans. Caused by misuse of prescription opioids, heroin, or other illicit opioids,[2] OUD carries with it significant mortality risks both from overdose risk and unrelated to overdose.[3] In 2021 alone, there were more than 75,000 overdose deaths attributed to opioids.[4]

Methadone, an opioid agonist, is one of the effective treatments for OUD . Methadone both lowers the likelihood of overdose and reduces illicit opioid use. However, a fairly narrow regulatory approach limits methadone access. Methadone currently may be dispensed for the treatment of OUD only in federally approved opioid treatment programs (OTPs).[1]

In this paper, the author considers efforts to facilitate access to methadone outside the traditional OTP delivery mechanisms for medications for OUD (MOUD). To this end, the objective of this scoping review was to identify treatment pilots or programs that (1) were delivered under regulations that differ from the traditionally applicable federal regulations or (2) offer new strategies or practices to OTPs within

---

[*] The author is responsible for the content of this article, which does not necessarily represent the views of the National Academies of Sciences, Engineering, and Medicine.

the parameters of the traditional federal regulations and to describe what evidence exists of their efficacy to inform future clinical and policy discussions regarding MOUD in the U.S. context.

RESULTS

Pandemic Response Results

The COVID-19 pandemic stimulated a regulatory effort to ease access to MOUD in the United States. The results of this review were classified into two categories: (1) innovations specifically brought about by or in response to the COVID-19 pandemic, and (2) innovations in methadone treatment prior to or not prompted by the pandemic. The author makes this distinction because the regulatory shifts made in response to the COVID-19 pandemic have allowed for new and different approaches to methadone medication not permitted earlier. Additionally, because some of these innovations were made possible only by regulatory flexibility induced by the COVID-19 pandemic, the evidence bearing on their impact is limited by its length.

The pandemic exacerbated the difficulties faced by people who use opioids. At the same time, it resulted in significant shifts in the regulatory landscape that normally governs methadone treatment. In March 2020, the Substance Abuse and Mental Health Services Administration (SAMHSA) allowed states to request a blanket exemption allowing OTPs to issue as many as 28 days' worth of take-home methadone for patients considered "stable" and 14 days for those considered "less stable," and the Drug Enforcement Administration (DEA) granted an exemption allowing alternate delivery protocols of medication.[5,6] In June 2021, DEA issued an exemption to the rules for certifying mobile medication units to allow OTPs an additional treatment pathway to reach their patients.[7] Additionally, the Centers for Medicare & Medicaid Services issued payment and reimbursement guidelines that allowed OTP reimbursement for MOUD treatment provided by telehealth under certain circumstances.[8] In this section, the author examines early evidence from methadone innovations introduced in response to the COVID-19 pandemic.

Telehealth and E-Health

Telehealth and e-health implemented for OUD treatment, where regulation allows, can include replacing in-person counseling for methadone or buprenorphine treatment programs with audio or audiovisual appointments, as well as prescribing MOUD electronically.[9] Data on the effects of allowing clinical oversight of telehealth patients receiving MOUD in OTPs are limited.

Programs across the country responded to this ease in regulation by implementing telemedicine at multiple points in the treatment pipeline, including the mandatory methadone counseling normally conducted in person at the OTP. Neither Chan and colleagues' recent scoping review of these changes, nor any of the studies identified in this review, demonstrated a significant difference in treatment retention or patient satisfaction, but most focused on a single clinic in their measurements.[10] Some providers have expressed concerns regarding retention and diversion when asked directly, which might demonstrate a need for better education about the merits of telehealth.[11] Provider concerns may be validated as more robust data become available, but there is not yet enough information to respond to these concerns. Chan and colleagues' review identified multiple studies where existing gaps in access to the Internet negatively impacted patient experience. In addition, this review notes that these disparities in digital access often reflect existing racial and ethnic disparities in quality of care, and may worsen them.[9]

In Rhode Island, one new telehealth MOUD counseling program demonstrated increased flexibility in provision of care by clinicians, higher patient retention rates, and more patient reports of access to care.[12] A Boston OUD center transitioned nearly all of its existing patient interactions to telehealth across multiple programs, with little to no retention issues across all programs, but their only reported MOUD program was for buprenorphine rather than methadone.[13]

At this stage, it is difficult to draw conclusions regarding tele-MOUD because of the limited data available, but the studies and case reports available suggest that telehealth may provide an opportunity for OTPs to increase access while maintaining retention.

Increased Take-Home Dosing

The effects of increased take-home dosing of methadone have become more clear as the pandemic has spread, but data are still limited because of the short period of time during which the federal changes have been in effect and the small number of studies conducted to date.

One of the first studies available on the impact of the new take-home rules on OTP behavior is a pre/post study conducted in Spokane, WA. This study demonstrated a rapid and marked uptick in take-home dosing following the regulatory easing, presumably in response to swift implementation by OTPs.[14] One concern often flagged regarding increased take-home dosing of methadone is the greater possibility of diversion, but the data thus far do not support that idea. Another Washington study, as well as studies in North Carolina and Spain, showed little to no detectable increase in diversion among their patients.[15,16,17] A qualitative assessment of the increase in take-home supply among rural methadone patients identified a sense of increased humanity (feeling "more like a regular person") and quality-of-life improvements in regaining access to time for work or with family that might have otherwise been spent at or traveling to a clinic.[18] A second concern about increased take-home dosing is greater opioid and non-opioid drug use, which was observed by Bart and colleagues. Despite that observed shift, their analysis indicated that this increase could not be attributed to the increase in take-home doses.[19]

In sum, although data are limited, studies conducted to date have not found any evidence of diversion or other adverse effects of expanding the take-home supply of methadone.

Separate from the analyses of take-home dosing, one study highlighted a potential technology-assisted intervention (an electronic pillbox) to assuage worries of diversion, finding in a small sample (25) that participants were satisfied and none of the pillbox users attempted to divert the medication.[20]

One final aspect of take-home dosing worth noting is that the shift may not have affected all patients equally. Harris and colleagues found that unhoused Boston patients reported that take-home adaptations exacerbated existing inequities for them–including limitations on take-home dosing for the unhoused and the increased social instability felt from virtual counseling– and recommended that any further take-home efforts should take into account those inequities when designing these adaptations.[21]

Innovations Unrelated to Pandemic Response

While the COVID-19 pandemic has provided a unique opportunity to observe the effects of changes to OTPs' delivery of methadone, it is not the lone source of innovations in methadone treatment. Pilot programs under the prepandemic regulatory framework and programs implemented outside the United States offer additional lessons on ways in which methods of methadone delivery affect patient outcomes.

Mobile Treatment and Outreach

Prior to a regulatory shift by DEA in 2007, mobile medication units were a permissible way to dispense methadone in rural communities and other hard-to-reach populations outside of a traditional OTP setting. In a scoping review of these programs, Chan, Hoffman and colleagues found no evidence that these programs significantly decreased treatment quality. Moreover, some evidence showed that (1) retention actually increased compared with fixed-site programs, and (2) mobile units in some cases made it easier to reach hard-to-treat populations.[22]

In addition to those mobile medication units, at least one OTP network (in Philadelphia) has established a mobile engagement unit (MEU) that provides free transportation to an OTP for intake (but not free transportation for ongoing treatment thereafter). Despite being only a one-time intervention, the study participants enrolled by the MEU showed statistically significant improvements in retention compared with other enrollees in MOUD at that OTP. The lack of randomization and limited scope of this intervention weaken the strength of these results, but this style of intervention may be worth studying at scale.[23]

Integrated Care Models

Because injection drug use is a method of transmission for HIV and the hepatitis C virus (HCV), clinicians have sought to improve MOUD retention and patient experience by integrating MOUD delivery with treatment for these viruses, as well as with syringe exchange programs (SEPs). Low and colleagues' systematic review of the literature on concurrent use of antiretroviral therapies (ARTs) and MOUD, including methadone, demonstrated significant increases in initiation of ART and viral suppression, as well as significant reduction in attrition rates.[24] Another review of these integrated HIV care models has shown the potential for reducing HIV transmission rates, though it is difficult to determine the extent to which that reduction in use resulted from MOUD treatment itself rather than the integration of ART and other HIV care with MOUD.[25]

While there is no systematic scoping review of the HCV and MOUD literature, a study of a program in Bronx, NY, that concurrently offered HCV treatment and methadone treatment showed promising results for potential treatment retention for both disorders and suggested concurrent treatment might be particularly apt for injection drug users who have demonstrated psychosocial vulnerability.[26] A New Haven, CT, study found that a full integration of HCV and MOUD services at an existing OTP was feasible and that program support from both clinicians and administrators was important for replicability.[27] Both of these studies are limited by their geographic scope and observation of only a single OTP in each case.

This review did not identify any integration efforts between SEPs and methadone treatment at the point of syringe exchange, but multiple studies considered the efficacy of SEP *referrals* compared with other pathways. Multiple studies identified in this scoping review demonstrate successful initiation into treatment from SEP referrals, but in the United States thus far those referrals have shown higher rates of attrition from treatment than other enrollment pathways.[28] One study in Sweden showed more effective rates of retention using similar methods, but with a small sample size (71 enrollees).[29]

Interim Methadone

McCarty, Chan, and colleagues. conducted a scoping review of "interim methadone" — which refers to the provision of methadone without counseling for up to 120 days when patient circumstances require. They found that interim methadone "is associated with reductions in waitlists, less delay in receiving medication, decreased drug use, and enhanced program retention with better outcomes than no care."[30] Despite those findings, interim methadone remains in limited use because of SAMHSA's specific authorization requirement, the lack of take-home dosing, and the restriction against its use by for-profit OTPs (which account for more than half of all currently operating OTPs in the United States).

Pharmacy-Based Methadone

Some methadone delivery strategies banned in the United States are permitted abroad. Pharmacy-based methadone — widely used in Canada, the United Kingdom, and Australia — is perhaps the most prominent among them. While some differences across countries exist, they share some basic features. A patient receives an initial assessment by a licensed medical professional; after that assessment, a prescription for MOUD is issued, and the local pharmacy dispenses MOUD doses, sometimes including supervision of the dosing. The initial prescriber may still provide additional care.[31] Although pharmacists participate at quite a high rate in the United Kingdom (e.g., 88 percent participation rate in Scotland), pharmacies in Australia have shown less willingness to offer MOUD.[32,33] Furthermore, while increased access, especially in rural areas, is a significant benefit of pharmacy-based distribution, at least one comparative study in Canada showed a more than 40 percent increase in retention for the more centralized treatment option over community pharmacy-based dispensing.[34] While such dispensing is a promising opportunity, this finding suggests that it should be implemented to take into account local context and patient needs.

The most significant potential advantage of pharmacy-based methadone in the United States is improved geographic access. A study of drive time in Appalachian areas showed that 6 percent of patients in the region faced a drive time of more than one hour to the nearest OTP, and that in rural areas, the median drive time to pharmacies was at least 30 minutes lower than the nearest OTP.[35] A recent clinical trial examined pharmacy-based methadone in the United States for both feasibility and acceptability and found pharmacy-based treatment both feasible and acceptable, with 80 percent retention at month 3 of the trial and 100 percent treatment adherence among those patients retained. That study's results are limited by the small patient count for this first trial, with only 20 patients enrolled.[36]

Office-Based Methadone

A scoping review of office-based methadone, delivering treatment in office settings like general practice or primary care, by McCarty and colleagues identified 18 studies of patients treated with office-based methadone, including observational and clinical studies. These studies were limited to only stable methadone patients, and consistently found patient value and treatment satisfaction for office-based care and treatment outcomes, including low rates of drug use, comparable to OTP care. A primary limitation on this literature is that none of the observational or clinical studies took place after 2010, and more contemporary study of the method in the United States would speak to the continued applicability of this model.[37]

Lessons from Non-Methadone MOUD

Methadone is not the only form of MOUD administered in the United States. Buprenorphine and buprenorphine combined with naloxone (also known as Suboxone) are offered in contexts where methadone is not — in large part due to the narrower authorization of methadone administration. While studies examining these drugs are thus not directly translatable to the methadone context, they still have some common features, most notably that the participating patients all are being treated for OUD.

One advantage of buprenorphine, as compared with current U.S. methadone administration, is the ability to prescribe and manage the medication in an office-based setting as compared to an OTP. A significant advantage of office-based treatment is increased access. A travel time analysis of the distance from office-based buprenorphine treatment, as compared to an OTP, showed that the gap between the two, especially in rural areas, was significant.[38]

As noted above, community pharmacies have significant potential to increase access to MOUD, especially in rural areas in the United States. Wu and colleagues conducted a pilot physician–pharmacist collaborative to take advantage of both community proximity and the respective treatment specialties of each party to demonstrate the feasibility of a collaborative care model. That pilot (71 participants) demonstrated significant retention and adherence, a further data point for the potential of increased reliance on community pharmacies in U.S. MOUD treatment.[39]

DISCUSSION

COVID-19 has provided a unique opportunity to examine the effects of a different regulatory landscape on methadone treatment in the United States. Although the data from the pandemic are limited, and surely will be augmented in the years ahead, early studies show a significant increase in take-home doses of methadone and suggest that increased flexibility for OTPs could yield dividends in both patient experience and treatment retention and adherence. More research is needed to increase confidence in that conclusion, especially given the lack of geographic diversity of the studies identified in this review. While telehealth undoubtedly provides certain advantages during a pandemic (e.g., decreased risk of viral transmission), its long-term impact on methadone treatment is not yet known. The regulatory flexibility that allowed these innovations is tied to the COVID-19 public health emergency declaration. For this reason, it is imperative that research be intensified to document their effects while the window remains open.

Beyond the pandemic, the literature reviewed identified challenges to MOUD access in rural areas. It highlighted the potential for leveraging existing institutions (e.g., community pharmacies) or common-sense interventions (e.g., transportation to intake) as opportunities to meet those challenges. Pharmacy-based delivery has become the norm in other countries, but multiple confounding variables prevent direct translation to the U.S. setting. The political, geographic, and cultural makeup of the United States is not that of the United Kingdom or Canada or Australia, so U.S.-centered pilot studies are needed to assess whether those findings would be replicated in the United States.

Lastly, integrated care models of methadone treatment offer opportunities to meet patients across multiple axes of care sometimes implicated by injection drug use. Integrated care has shown promise regarding the ability of MOUD to improve care for HIV or hepatitis C, as well as for the associated OUD.

REFERENCES

1. Substance Abuse and Mental Health Services Administration. *Medications for Opioid Use Disorder*. Published online 2021.

2. Committee on Medication-Assisted Treatment for Opioid Use Disorder, Board on Health Sciences Policy, Health and Medicine Division, National Academies of Sciences, Engineering, and Medicine. *Medications for opioid use disorder save lives.* (Leshner AI, Mancher M, eds.). The National Academies Press; 2019:25310. doi:10.17226/25310

3. Bahji A, Cheng B, Gray S, Stuart H. Mortality among people with opioid use disorder: A systematic review and meta-analysis. *Journal of Addiction Medicine*. 2020;14(4):e118-e132. doi:10.1097/ADM.0000000000000606

4. Ahmad F, Rossen L, Sutton P. Provisional drug overdose death counts. *National Center for Health Statistics*. Published online 2022.

5. SAMHSA. *Methadone Take-Home Flexibilities Extension Guidance*. Accessed February 18, 2022. https://www.samhsa.gov/medication-assisted-treatment/statutes-regulations-guidelines/methadone-guidance

6. McDermott WT. Published online March 16, 2020. https://www.deadiversion.usdoj.gov/GDP/(DEA-DC-015)%20SAMHSA%20Exemption%20NTP%20Deliveries%20(CoronaVirus).pdf

7. *Registration Requirements for Narcotic Treatment Programs With Mobile Components*; 2021. https://www.deadiversion.usdoj.gov/fed_regs/rules/2021/fr0628_3.pdf

8. *Opioid Treatment Programs (OTPs) Medicare Billing & Payment*. Centers for Medicare & Medicaid Services; 2021.

9. Krawczyk N, Fawole A, Yang J, Tofighi B. Early innovations in opioid use disorder treatment and harm reduction during the COVID-19 pandemic: A scoping review. *Addiction Science & Clinical Practice*. 2021;16(1):68. doi:10.1186/s13722-021-00275-1

10. Uscher-Pines L, Raja P, Mehrotra A, Huskamp HA. Health center implementation of telemedicine for opioid use disorders: A qualitative assessment of adopters and nonadopters. *Journal of Substance Abuse Treatment*. 2020;115:108037. doi:10.1016/j.jsat.2020.108037

11. Chan B, Bougatsos C, Priest KC, McCarty D, Grusing S, Chou R. Opioid treatment programs, telemedicine and COVID-19: A scoping review. *Substance Abuse*. 2022;43(1):539-546. doi:10.1080/08897077.2021.1967836

12. Hughto JMW, Peterson L, Perry NS, et al. The provision of counseling to patients receiving medications for opioid use disorder: Telehealth innovations and challenges in the age of COVID-19. *Journal of Substance Abuse Treatment*. 2021;120:108163. doi:10.1016/j.jsat.2020.108163

13. Komaromy M, Tomanovich M, Taylor JL, et al. Adaptation of a system of treatment for substance use disorders during the COVID-19 pandemic. *Journal of Addiction Medicine*. 2021;15(6):448-451. doi:10.1097/ADM.0000000000000791

14. Amram O, Amiri S, Thorn EL, Lutz R, Joudrey PJ. Changes in methadone take-home dosing before and after COVID-19. *Journal of Substance Abuse Treatment*. Published online June 2021:108552. doi:10.1016/j.jsat.2021.108552

15. Amram O, Amiri S, Panwala V, Lutz R, Joudrey PJ, Socias E. The impact of relaxation of methadone take-home protocols on treatment outcomes in the COVID-19 era. *The American Journal of Drug and Alcohol Abuse*. 2021;47(6):722-729. doi:10.1080/00952990.2021.1979991

16. Trujols J, Larrabeiti A, Sànchez O, Madrid M, De Andrés S, Duran-Sindreu S. Increased flexibility in methadone take-home scheduling during the COVID-19 pandemic: Should this practice be incorporated into routine clinical care? *Journal of Substance Abuse Treatment*. 2020;119:108154. doi:10.1016/j.jsat.2020.108154

17. Figgatt MC, Salazar Z, Day E, Vincent L, Dasgupta N. Take-home dosing experiences among persons receiving methadone maintenance treatment during COVID-19. *Journal of Substance Abuse Treatment*. 2021;123:108276. doi:10.1016/j.jsat.2021.108276

18. Levander XA, Hoffman KA, McIlveen JW, McCarty D, Terashima JP, Korthuis PT. Rural opioid treatment program patient perspectives on take-home methadone policy changes

during COVID-19: A qualitative thematic analysis. *Addiction Science & Clinical Practice.* 2021;16(1):72. doi:10.1186/s13722-021-00281-3

19. Bart G, Wastvedt S, Hodges JS, Rosenthal R. Did drug use increase following COVID-19 relaxation of methadone take-out regulations? 2020 was a complicated year. *Journal of Substance Abuse Treatment.* 2022;133:108590. doi:10.1016/j.jsat.2021.108590

20. Dunn KE, Brooner RK, Stoller KB. Technology-assisted methadone take-home dosing for dispensing methadone to persons with opioid use disorder during the COVID-19 pandemic. *Journal of Substance Abuse Treatment.* 2021;121:108197. doi:10.1016/j.jsat.2020.108197

21. Harris MTH, Lambert AM, Maschke AD, Bagley SM, Walley AY, Gunn CM. "No home to take methadone to": Experiences with addiction services during the COVID-19 pandemic among survivors of opioid overdose in Boston. *Journal of Substance Abuse Treatment.* Published online November 2021:108655. doi:10.1016/j.jsat.2021.108655

22. Chan B, Hoffman KA, Bougatsos C, Grusing S, Chou R, McCarty D. Mobile methadone medication units: A brief history, scoping review and research opportunity. *Journal of Substance Abuse Treatment.* 2021;129:108483. doi:10.1016/j.jsat.2021.108483

23. Stewart RE, Shen L, Kwon N, et al. Transporting to treatment: Evaluating the effectiveness of a mobile engagement unit. *Journal of Substance Abuse Treatment.* 2021;129:108377. doi:10.1016/j.jsat.2021.108377

24. Low AJ, Mburu G, Welton NJ, et al. Impact of opioid substitution therapy on antiretroviral therapy outcomes: A systematic review and meta-analysis. *Clinical Infectious Diseases.* 2016;63(8):1094-1104. doi:10.1093/cid/ciw416

25. MacArthur GJ, Minozzi S, Martin N, et al. Opiate substitution treatment and HIV transmission in people who inject drugs: Systematic review and meta-analysis. *BMJ.* 2012;345(oct03 3):e5945-e5945. doi:10.1136/bmj.e5945

26. Stein MR, Soloway IJ, Jefferson KS, Roose RJ, Arnsten JH, Litwin AH. Concurrent group treatment for hepatitis C: Implementation and outcomes in a methadone maintenance treatment program. *Journal of Substance Abuse Treatment.* 2012;43(4):424-432. doi:10.1016/j.jsat.2012.08.007

27. Bruce RD, Eiserman J, Acosta A, Gote C, Lim JK, Altice FL. Developing a modified directly observed therapy intervention for hepatitis C treatment in a methadone maintenance program: Implications for program replication. *The American Journal of Drug and Alcohol Abuse.* 2012;38(3):206-212. doi:10.3109/00952990.2011.643975

28. Kidorf M, Brooner RK, Leoutsakos JM, Peirce J. Reducing risky drug use behaviors by enrolling syringe exchange registrants in methadone maintenance. *Substance Use & Misuse.* 2021;56(4):546-551. doi:10.1080/10826084.2021.1887253

29. Bråbäck M, Ekström L, Troberg K, et al. Malmö Treatment Referral and Intervention Study — High 12-month retention rates in patients referred from syringe exchange to methadone or

buprenorphine/naloxone treatment. *Front Psychiatry*. 2017;8:161. doi:10.3389/fpsyt.2017.00161

30. McCarty D, Chan B, Bougatsos C, Grusing S, Chou R. Interim methadone – Effective but underutilized: A scoping review. *Drug and Alcohol Dependence*. 2021;225:108766. doi:10.1016/j.drugalcdep.2021.108766

31. Cochran G, Bruneau J, Cox N, Gordon AJ. Medication treatment for opioid use disorder and community pharmacy: Expanding care during a national epidemic and global pandemic. *Substance Abuse*. 2020;41(3):269-274. doi:10.1080/08897077.2020.1787300

32. Matheson C, Thiruvothiyur M, Robertson H, Bond C. Community pharmacy services for people with drug problems over two decades in Scotland: Implications for future development. *International Journal of Drug Policy*. 2016;27:105-112. doi:10.1016/j.drugpo.2015.11.006

33. Chaar B. Provision of opioid substitution therapy services in Australian pharmacies. *AMJ*. 2011;4(4):210-216. doi:10.4066/AMJ.2011.706

34. Gauthier G, Eibl JK, Marsh DC. Improved treatment-retention for patients receiving methadone dosing within the clinic providing physician and other health services (onsite) versus dosing at community (offsite) pharmacies. *Drug and Alcohol Dependence*. 2018;191:1-5. doi:10.1016/j.drugalcdep.2018.04.029

35. Joudrey PJ, Chadi N, Roy P, et al. Pharmacy-based methadone dispensing and drive time to methadone treatment in five states within the United States: A cross-sectional study. *Drug and Alcohol Dependence*. 2020;211:107968. doi:10.1016/j.drugalcdep.2020.107968

36. Wu L, John WS, Morse ED, et al. Opioid treatment program and community pharmacy collaboration for methadone maintenance treatment: Results from a feasibility clinical trial. *Addiction*. 2022;117(2):444-456. doi:10.1111/add.15641

37. McCarty D, Bougatsos C, Chan B, et al. Office-based methadone treatment for opioid use disorder and pharmacy dispensing: A scoping review. *AJP*. 2021;178(9):804-817. doi:10.1176/appi.ajp.2021.20101548

38. Wu L, John WS, Ghitza UE, et al. Buprenorphine physician–pharmacist collaboration in the management of patients with opioid use disorder: Results from a multisite study of the National Drug Abuse Treatment Clinical Trials Network. *Addiction*. 2021;116(7):1805-1816. doi:10.1111/add.15353